Fundamental Aspects of Transcultural Nursing

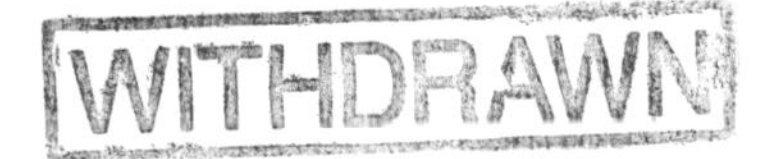

Fundamental Aspects of Transcultural Nursing

by
Sue Dyson

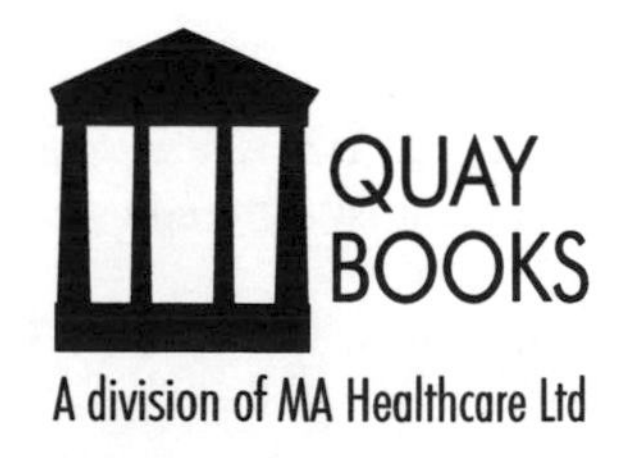

A division of MA Healthcare Ltd

Quay Books Division, MA Healthcare Ltd, St Jude's Church, Dulwich Road, London
SE24 0PB

British Library Cataloguing-in-Publication Data
A catalogue record is available for this book

ISBN-10: 1 85642 304 2 ISBN-13: 978 1 85642 304 5

Printed by Athenaeum Press Ltd, Dukes Way, Team Valley, Gateshead, NE11 OPZ

Contents

Acknowledgements

I would like to thank all nurses who constantly strive to provide the best possible care to patients and clients in multicultural Britain in what is often less than ideal situations, and often in the face of a great deal of criticism. This book recognises that nurses, at all times, do the best they can with the knowledge and skills they have. I would like to thank all those involved in nurse education as they strive to increase the transcultural knowledge of student nurses and practising nurses through education and training. This book recognises that in order to move the art and science of transcultural nursing forward we must learn together and avoid reverting to ethnocentrism in our learning and teaching and in our practice of transcultural care.

I thank my husband Simon, for his wisdom, academic prowess and constant support. His alternative perspective on life and his ability to see the point of view of the other person has helped shape this book. I thank both my step-children – Rehana, for showing us what it means to not quite be part of this world (if you don't read *this* book Rehana, please read *a* book); and Ingrid, for ensuring that when you think you have encountered all life has to offer, you haven't seen anything until you get step-children. Finally, I would like to thank Emma and Matt for their unconditional love and support despite my endless mistakes in life. They continually remind me that the world is not a perfect place and that it is okay to be less than perfect as a mother. Most people do the best they can with the knowledge they had at the time. Without mistakes, no learning can take place.

Sue Dyson 2007

Introduction

The art and science of transcultural nursing owes much to the work of Madeleine Leininger, considered by many to be a pioneer in the field. Leininger began her work in the mid 1950s in the USA on recognising a marked increase in cultural diversity and a trend towards globalisation. This, she argued, necessitated a new field of nursing care, namely transcultural nursing, not confined to the USA, but worldwide (Leininger, 1995). Since then the theory and practice of transcultural nursing has developed in many countries, albeit slowly, as a response to the global increase in cultural diversity resulting from the mass migration of people due to war, famine, disease, poverty, and the promise of a better life in another country.

In the UK, Professor Irena Papadopoulos became interested in transcultural nursing care when working as a community nurse in a particularly deprived multicultural area of London. She describes the frustration of being unable to communicate with patients who did not speak English and whose living conditions were often poor and overcrowded but who chose to ignore received wisdom in favour of using traditional unscientific ways to treat illnesses (Papadopoulos, 2002). This experience taught Papadopoulos the importance of respecting the wishes of individuals, of taking their views into consideration, modifying care to suit their needs, and linking with other agencies. However – perhaps more importantly – the experience led Papadopoulos to recognise her limitations in nursing in a culturally diverse society stemming from inadequate preparation during nurse training. Since the early 1980s Papadopoulos has worked in nurse education, focusing her energy on changing what she perceived to be a culturally blind curriculum.

In a similar fashion Kate Gerrish, Professor in Nursing Practice Development at the University of Sheffield, has worked for a number of years in the field of transcultural nursing with a special interest in transcultural competence. In the late 1990s she undertook a major study commissioned by the English National Board for Nursing, Midwifery and Health Visiting which examined the extent to which nurses and midwives were prepared to work in a multiethnic society. Gerrish (1997) concluded that while recognition of distinct cultural beliefs, customs and values is essential to providing appropriate care, these were not always adequately addressed in the nursing curriculum. Furthermore, while the opportunity to learn about different cultural perspectives was highly valued by students, teachers and practitioners participating in the study, by concentrating on the beliefs and practices of particular communities there is a risk of developing ethnic stereotypes which fails to take account of the diversity that exists both within and across ethnic communities. More recently a study by Narayanasamy (2003) explored how nurses responded to the cultural needs of their patients/clients. He found that while many nurses claimed they responded to the cultural needs of patients and that their clients' cultural needs were adequately met, further education in meeting cultural needs was needed.

Clearly, authors concerned with the field of transcultural nursing highlight the need to enhance the education of nurses working with clients from a diverse multiethnic society. This view is embedded in the Quality Assurance Agency for Higher Education's benchmark statement for nursing, which lists the knowledge, understanding and associated skills that are specific to nursing, including an understanding of anti-discriminatory practice, encompassing fairness, social inclusion, 'race' and culture (Quality Assurance Agency, 2001).

With this in mind, this book is designed to provide a foundation to the theory and practice of transcultural nursing. It will therefore be of use to students beginning to study nursing at undergraduate level and to practising nurses who are providing care to patients from an increasingly diverse society. It is not intended as a comprehensive account of different cultural groups, however, where appropriate, it draws on cultural knowledge to underpin a transcultural assessment. In addition, this book provides transcultural nursing knowledge that is applicable in cross-cultural transactions. In doing so, students and qualified practitioners will acquire a sound knowledge base from which to develop generic cultural competency as a prerequisite to the development of specific cultural competency. The book concludes with information on how transcultural nursing can be incorporated into the nursing curriculum and will be of use to nurse educators involved in planning and delivering transcultural nursing education.

Chapter One introduces the context, considers the changing nature of society and the demands placed on nurses to meets the needs of a multicultural population. A number of approaches to transcultural care have predominated in the UK over the past five decades, consistent with the history of and patterns of migration. These are considered as an explanation of emerging trends in transcultural nursing.

Chapter Two considers the theoretical underpinnings of transcultural nursing, including the use of appropriate language, race, ethnicity, human rights, multicultural health-care provision and emerging models of cultural competency. The chapter identifies the principles of good practice in relation to transcultural nursing.

Chapters Three, Four, Five and *Six* explore aspects of transcultural nursing that relate to the care of adults, children, and clients with mental health needs and with learning disabilities. The intention of this chapter is not to advocate a particular model of transcultural nursing; rather the reader is encouraged to reflect on the knowledge provided and to apply the principles of good practice in transcultural nursing within the framework of a preferred model. Please note that the detailed explanations of the ethnic culture within each case study are variable in scope and depth; in some cases diet is considered at length, and in other cases more attention is paid to economic factors. The reason for is that only certain cultural differences have relevance to the specifics of each case study covered, depending on a specific place, time, and social and medical history – to cover equally all aspects of these cultures in each case would be pointless for the purposes of this exercise.

Chapter Seven draws together and summarises considerations for undertaking a transcultural nursing assessment. It then addresses issues for nurse educators when planning how to incorporate transcultural education into the nursing curriculum. Guidance is offered to nurse educators who have responsibility for ensuring that nurses are capable of caring for patients, clients and carers from an increasingly diverse society and in increasingly complex and varied situations.

This book is written by a White English person – a former nurse and now university lecturer. As such, this means that the perspective of what it is like to practice as nurse in the UK as someone from a minority ethnic background in a multiethnic society (and, for example, to have to respond to the racism of some patients/clients, carers and staff) is not addressed in this book. But the work of learning how to nurse people from diverse backgrounds is the task of all nurses, from whatever background they themselves come. We cannot simply say that it is the responsibility of minority ethnic nurses to deal with transcultural issues. It is up to all of us to try to learn and develop. This means stepping outside of your comfort zone and taking risks.

In the area of ethnicity, the reader should know that there is no widespread agreement, even about the terms that are used, and so it is very easy to offend where offence is not intended. The important thing is to own the mistake when someone points this out, and to recognise and act on the changes to nursing practice required. Similarly, the terms patient and client may mean different things to different people in different contexts. Much debate is to be had regarding when and where to use these terms. In this book the term patient is used to denote a person in receipt of health care services for physical conditions, whereas the term client is used in cases where individuals are receiving health care related for mental health and learning difficulties.

CHAPTER 1

Transcultural Care In Context

Great Britain is traditionally a country of immigration and of emigration. As such, the British population is the result of the ethnic and cultural intermixture of successive influxes of migrants with those migrants already present. Furthermore, it is well recognised that Great Britain has benefited considerably, in economic and cultural terms, as a result of this tradition, especially from the post-war immigration from the New Commonwealth (all commonwealth countries excluding Australia, Canada, South Africa, and New Zealand) (Glover and Bellwood, 2004). To fully understand the cultural context of present-day Britain it is important to know something of the history of migration to these shores. An understanding of our cultural heritage enables us to understand better the perspectives of the people we will be caring for in a multiethnic Britain.

Historical perspectives on migration to Great Britain

The Romans

Historically, the Britain Isles has seen migration, albeit in relatively small numbers, from many countries for more than 2000 years. Between AD 43 and AD 411, the period when Britain was part of the Roman Empire, people came from all over the world as soldiers, merchants and administrators. During this time Great Britain drew its migrants from France, Germany and Eastern Europe. In May of AD 43, the Romans invaded Britain via France. Four legions and about 20 000 auxiliary troops landed on the Kent coast and defeated the Britons in a series of battles. In the autumn, Emperor Claudius arrived and supervised the capture of Colchester. Claudius accepted the surrender of eleven tribal kings, appointed the first Roman Governor of Britain, and returned to Rome. However, conflict did not end there; it continued between several British tribes and the Roman invaders. Some tribes – such as the Icenig (modern East Anglia), Atrebates (modern Sussex) and Brigantes (of northern 'England') quickly accepted Roman influence. Indeed, Fryer (1984) suggests that the Roman conquering battalions included those of African descent. Perhaps this was the beginnings of multiethnic Britain.

By AD 47, the Roman legions had penetrated as far south-west as Cornwall, as far west as Wales, and as far north as the Humber. The Romans began constructing a system of military roads, founded Londinium (modern London) and built a crossing over the river Thames. By AD 60, the frontier had been pushed further and more tribes had been taken under Roman 'protection'. By AD 410, Roman troops were being continually withdrawn from Britain to help with conflicts elsewhere in the Empire. Written and archaeological evidence from that period suggest that Romanised life in Britain continued well into the fifth century.

The Angles, Saxons, Jutes, Vikings and Normans

Angles (from the modern-day Denmark–Germany border), Saxons (from Germany), Jutes (from Denmark), and Vikings (from Scandinavia) followed with the last conquering invaders, the Normans, claiming the crown of England in 1066 under William the Conqueror. Effects of the conquest included a complete change of the ruling classes in English society: only thirteen English magnates can be found in the Domesday Book and French replaced English as the official language. These early settlers left their mark on Great Britain through religion, language, methods of farming, trade and road systems (Kershen, 2005).

Huguenot, Jewish and African migrations

Huguenots were French Protestants who fled Catholic persecution and moved to England during the sixteenth, seventeenth, and eighteenth centuries. Their main areas of settlement initially included towns such as Norwich and Canterbury. However, most of them settled eventually in areas of East London, such as Spitalfields, and the west end of London such as Soho. The expertise and skills of these settlers to Great Britain is still evident today, for example in manufacture of clocks and scientific instruments. Others were skilled at weaving silk and velvet, and their expertise helped to expand the weaving industry. During the eighteenth century members of the Huguenot and Jewish communities are recorded as giving major financial support to the state and the army.

The first Jewish settlers arrived in England after the Norman Conquest. However, most of these early Jewish immigrants were expelled in 1290 by King Edward I. Jewish migrants then settled in England following the English Civil War in 1646. The majority of Jews in the UK today are descendants from two periods of immigration by Ashkenazi Jews – Jews of central and eastern European origin. Ashkenazi Jews sought asylum in England between 1881 and 1914, and from 1933 onwards during the Nazi persecution in Germany. The 1905 Aliens Act was an early piece of anti-immigration legislation aimed specifically against Jewish migration. Since 1956 small numbers have arrived from Israel and Arab and eastern European countries.

Chinese, Irish, German and Italian migrations

The immigration of other peoples to the Britain Isles kept pace with the development of the British Empire, in that trade brought seamen from China, West Africa, and those countries known today as Somalia and the Yemen. Some of these travellers returned home, but others stayed and formed communities in port cities such as London and Liverpool, which today have well-established Chinese communities, as do a number of other cities in Britain.

The immigration of Irish labourers is well recorded. At the height of the industrial revolution in the first half of the nineteenth century, Irish labourers were drawn to build the roads, railways and canals needed to improve the transport of goods between the docks, the centres of manufacture, and shops in towns and cities around the country. Irish women immigrants came at the same time to work as domestics, and Irish children worked as street vendors. From the mid-nineteenth century German clerks came to the UK, attracted by higher wages. Their ability to speak English made them very employable.

Later in the nineteenth century, Italian people migrated to the British Isles and introduced the idea of street vending of ice-cream. They worked in catering, baking, confectionery and became café owners. Later, in the 1940s and 1950s, Italian men and women were drawn to work in factories and some went on to open restaurants and pizzerias (Kershen, 2005).

Migration during the First and Second World Wars

During both the First and Second World Wars, members of the British Empire throughout the world came to Great Britain to serve on merchant ships or in the forces. The First World War saw approximately 15 000 Caribbean men recruited into the British West Indies Regiment. Many people from the Caribbean were attracted to the work opportunities in munitions and chemical factories in various parts of Britain, especially the North West. The Second World War also saw large numbers of people from the Caribbean arriving in Britain, mostly to be nurses or, again, to join the armed forces. By the end of the war, a large number of Caribbean people were familiar with working life in Britain. The soldiers, sailors, and airmen who had served with the Allied Forces in Europe were eager to return to Britain following demobilisation and a few hundred left Jamaica. The most famous account of these events is the journey of the ship the *SS Empire Windrush*. However, this was by no means the only boat to leaves the shores of Jamaica for a new life in Britain. Andrea Levy's *Small Island* is interesting reading (Levy, 2004).

Migration in the post-War years

Other migrants from the Caribbean followed throughout the 1950s. Some of the Caribbean migrants became nurses and experienced racism throughout their working lives in Great Britain, but they nonetheless contributed enormously to the success of the National Health Service (Culley *et al*, 2001). Migration from the Indian sub-continent (modern-day India, Pakistan, Bangladesh and Sri Lanka, ie. those of South Asian descent) also took place after the Second World War, and filled labour shortages in low-paid factory and industrial work, especially in woollens and textiles. Historically, students have travelled to Britain to study at university, mostly in law or medicine. While most of these students returned home, some chose to stay and settle after qualifying, particularly Indian doctors. In the 1960s and early 1970s, people of South Asian descent also came to Britain from East Africa. Their ancestors had been recruited by the British Empire to work in colonial administration in Africa, and also to work on the African railways. With the independence of a number of these East African countries from Britain, movements for the 're-Africanisation of Africa' turned some Africans against the British Asians, who were encouraged or forced to leave. It is important to recognise that those who migrated from the Indian sub-continent and those who migrated from East Africa represent diverse geographical origins, languages, ethnic groups and religions.

The diversity within British Asian communities is reflected by variation in geographical origins, as summarised below:

Origins in India
- Punjab State – Sikh and Hindu
- Gujarat State – Hindu and Muslim
- The Kutch (part of the Gujarat) – Muslim and Hindu

Origins in Pakistan
- North-west frontier area – Pathan peoples, Muslim, speak Pashto
- Mirpur border area – Mirpur peoples, Muslim, speak Mirpuri
- Kashmir, in which Muslims are a majority (a disputed territory in that some people want it to be part of India, some to be part of Pakistan, and others want independence)
- Province of Punjab – Punjabi peoples, Muslim, speak Punjabi and Urdu

Origins in Bangladesh
- Sylhet (North-east Bangladesh) border area – Muslim
- Maritime East India area – Muslim

Origins in East Africa
- Uganda
- Kenya
- Tanzania
- Malawi
- Zambia

Late twentieth-century migration

Although Great Britain continued to receive migrants throughout the twentieth century, the emigration rate often exceeded the immigration rate. Other groups to settle included the Vietnamese from 1975 onwards. These were 'ethnic' Chinese people living in Vietnam who had supported the USA and South Vietnam but who fled to Hong Kong with the defeat of the US army in the Vietnam War. A number of wars displaced peoples from (among other places) Somalia, Bosnia, Kosovo, Iraq, Sierra Leone and the Democratic People's Republic of the Congo in the last decades of the twentieth century. The political regime of Robert Mugabe and the economic crisis in Zimbabwe also led to a number of Zimbabweans coming to the UK, some of whom trained as nurses.

There are a great many myths about migrants, asylum seekers and refugees. Given that it is one of the richest countries in the world, the UK does not receive a large proportion of refugees. In 2002, Britain was home to less than 3% of the world's asylum seekers and refugees. Neither Africa nor the Indian sub-continent provides the largest migrant groups. About 8% of the British population was born abroad. Of these, 31% came from other European countries, 19% from Africa, 20% from the Indian sub-continent and 11% from the Americas, including Canada, the USA and the Caribbean (Home Office, 2002b). Furthermore, migrants to the UK do not use up resources but have a net positive effect on the economy. Research by the British government estimated that in 1999–2000 migrants contributed £31.2 billion in taxes and consumed £28.8 billion in benefits and state services, which means that they made an overall contribution of approximately £2.5 billion. This figure is equivalent to a 1% decrease in the basic rate of income tax (Home Office, 2002a).

Key dates in the history of multiethnic Britain during the twentieth-century

1905 The Aliens Act 1905 attempts to restrict Jewish immigration

1919 The Black community in Liverpool and Cardiff is subjected to physical attacks

1925 The Special Restrictions (Coloured Alien Seamen) Order prohibits Black British sailors from working on British ships and forces many of them out of the country

1938 *Kristallnacht* in Nazi Germany prompts new Jewish emigration

1945 2.5 million Indian soldiers fight for Great Britain in the Second World War

1948 The British Nationality Act confirms the right of those in Commonwealth countries to come to Britain with their families to work and to settle

1955 Recruitment drives are held in the Caribbean by British Transport, British Hotels and Restaurants Association, and the National Health Service

1958 Black communities in Nottingham and in Notting Hill, Kensal, Notting Dale and Paddington are subjected to physical attacks and petrol bombings during anti-Black riots

1962 The Commonwealth Immigrants Act restricts the right of Commonwealth citizens to come to Great Britain. It transforms temporary migration to permanent migration as immigration rates peak (people take the last opportunity to exercise their legal right of settlement that the act takes away)

1965 Race Relations Act creates a 'Race Relations Board' and Conciliation Committees

1966 Section 11 of the Local Government Act creates a source of money to support 'immigrants'

1968 Introduction of the Commonwealth Immigrants Act. The Labour government establishes quotas for British Asian citizens, resident in East Africa (Kenya, Tanzania, Uganda, Malawi and Zambia) restricting the right of these British citizens to come to the UK

1971 The Immigration Act ends so-called 'primary' immigration into the UK. It sets up two new terms 'patrial' and 'non-patrial' that refer to parents or grandparents born in the UK. In this way the Act effectively permits 'White immigration' from Australia, Canada, New Zealand and South Africa ('Old Commonwealth'), but restricts 'Black immigration' from Africa, the Caribbean and the Indian sub-continent ('New Commonwealth')

1972 The Ugandan dictator Idi Amin expels Ugandan Asians at short notice. Many lose their businesses and homes and are robbed of their personal possessions on the way to the airport. They then face further discrimination when they arrive in the UK

1976 The Labour government introduces the Race Relations Act. The Community Relations Commission and the Race Relations Board are replaced by the Commission for Racial Equality. The Act makes it unlawful to discriminate directly or indirectly against anyone 'on racial grounds' and prohibits discrimination by way of victimisation in the areas of employment, education, training and housing

1981 The British Nationality Act abolishes the automatic right of someone born on British soil to British citizenship

1983 The 'Primary Purpose' rule excludes many South-Asian husbands of British women from entering the UK

1985 The European Court of Human Rights rules that British immigration law is discriminatory against women. The government responds by making the law equally restrictive for men

1988 The Immigration Act removes the last remaining rights under British law for Commonwealth men to be joined by their wives in Great Britain. It also restricts the right of appeal against deportation

1993 The Black teenager Stephen Lawrence is murdered at a south London bus-stop

1994 The Criminal Justice and Public Order Act repeals the 1968 Caravans Sites Act removing the duty (which few had ever properly fulfilled) on local authorities to provide sites, and abolishing the government grant for constructing Gypsy caravan sites

1999 Publication of the *Macpherson Report* about the death of Stephen Lawrence brings the phrase 'institutional racism' into wider usage

2000 The Labour government passes the Race Relations (Amendment) Act. This Act extends the scope of the 1976 Act to outlaw acts of discrimination in all other public functions carried out by public bodies. The Act also places a general duty on public authorities to work towards the elimination of unlawful discrimination and to promote equality of opportunity and good relations between persons of different racial groups in the carrying out of their functions

Emerging trends in transcultural nursing

As the preceding discussion shows, Great Britain has always received migrants on its shores, from many different countries. Culturally diverse Britain owes much to its history and it is clear the process of industrialisation and the advent of war and its aftermath gave rise to momentous patterns of migration and immigration to fulfil shortfalls in labour and to support the economy. However, it is clear that members of our multicultural society have not enjoyed fair treatment, nor had their human rights respected in a way that is equitable with people who might lay claim to be the indigenous population of Britain – a tenuous claim given its history.

Papadopoulos (2006) identifies a number of emerging trends that over the decades have sought to enhance harmony in a culturally diverse Britain. She writes that during the 1950s and 1960s the approach was one of assimilation, in which members of minority cultural groups were encouraged to take on the values of the society in which they found themselves. Migrants were encouraged to believe that to have distinct cultural identities would be detrimental to their health and well being. This approach is not dissimilar to the adage 'When in Rome do as the Romans do'. However, the result of this 'assimilation' approach was a loss of distinctiveness. Recent empirical research with Zimbabwean nursing students currently living and studying in Britain shows that assimilation is still expected if students are to integrate into

British culture. It is evident that some working practices discourage cultural individuality, for example, visa requirements whereby only full-time study followed by full-time working is permitted in order that visa entitlement is not breached. African cultures naturally place a high value on family ties and relationships and for many African students working and studying full time is at odds with their cultural identity (Dyson, 2005a).

Of the 1970s and early 1980s Papadopoulos writes about 'multiculturalism', in which the promotion of understanding of each others' cultures reduces unfounded fears of the majority cultural group, while at the same time helping the minority cultural group to adapt to their adopted country. The thinking behind this approach is one of a gradual acceptance of diversity and the acknowledgement that through better understanding and prolonged contact between cultural groups, the migrant groups will incorporate the values and behaviours of the host culture. Papadopoulos describes this process as one of 'acculturation', whereby the host culture learns to accept cultural differences. Culley and Dyson (2001) describe the central aim of multiculturalism during this period as seeking to challenge the idea of 'ethnic' cultural difference in favour of a pluralistic society within which distinct ethnic communities reside in mutual harmony, understanding and acceptance. While this might at first appear hopeful as a way forward, it assumes, in fact, a position of dominance of the so-called host culture as one which the migrant culture would necessarily want to adopt in the place of their particular cultural identity. In addition, it is based on the assumption that it is possible for a common set of stable cultural characteristics to exist.

In the 1980s and early 1990s, the anti-racist movement dominated as an alternative response to multiculturalism. The anti-racist movement argued that the inequalities experienced by people from minority ethnic groups was due to racist polices and structures within society, as well as the racist attitudes of the majority group. Papadopoulos writes that these attitudes have their roots in the domination by British colonialists of many of the countries from which migrant communities are drawn. Interestingly, African nursing students who recounted experiences of racism still refer to Great Britain as the 'mother country' and a country that they believe themselves entitled to be part of (Dyson, 2005a).

From the mid-1990s a new combined approach of multiculturalism and anti-racism was in evidence, with an emphasis on the promotion of equality and citizenship. This new way of thinking recognised that the interests of people are not dictated by any one single factor. Multiple factors play a part in the way a person experiences the world. Age, gender and class, as well as race, determine the nature of a person's experience.

Conclusions

In conclusion, this chapter has considered the history of multicultural Britain. Patterns of migration have been discussed in order to show that today's ethnically diverse Britain is as much a result of an historical drive for superiority and dominance as it is a result of an effort to become industrialised and so to prosper. In spite of increasing diversity it is clear that many ethnic groups in the UK have not enjoyed fair and equitable treatment when compared to their White British counterparts. Over the last five decades a number of different approaches have been taken towards promoting harmony, fairness and equality within our diverse society. These approaches include assimilation, multiculturalism, anti-racism and a combined approach of anti-racism and multiculturalism. However, recent empirical evidence suggests that some elements of those outdated ways of thinking prevail. It is fair to say that members of minority ethnic groups are still expected to 'sign up to' the culture of their adopted country if their life is to be in any way acceptable. The ability of a particular cultural group to assimilate may be indicative of the level of tension experienced by that group. It seems clear that efforts to think in new ways in relation to transcultural care have been thwarted in recent years. An inability to engage with other cultures, fuelled by lack of understanding, has led to a rise in racial tension. It is also important to recognise that most people who draw upon cultures that differ from that of the nurse's will themselves have been born in Britain. It is, therefore, one of the most insulting questions to ask where a patient/client is 'from' because most minority ethnic individual will have been born and raised in the UK.

For practising nurses and student nurses working in an ethnically diverse Britain, the need to be knowledgeable in transcultural care and thus move towards cultural competency in caring for patients/clients from many different ethnic groups is paramount. The next chapter discusses key concepts in transcultural nursing.

CHAPTER 2

Key Concepts in Transcultural Nursing

Over recent years there has been a growing interest in the nursing care of patients/clients from minority ethnic communities. This includes the provision of nursing care and the training of health-care professionals to provide care for individuals from a diverse range of minority ethnic groups (Serrant-Green, 2001). The impetus for the promotion of transcultural competence and the development of the specific skills required by nurses to ensure the provision of high-quality and appropriate care within a multiethnic society stems from a number of issues, namely changes in the demography of the UK and the government's response to this over the last four years. The government's response involves a policy shift from addressing ethnic variations in health to focusing on inequalities in health and managing diversity (Papadopoulos and Lees, 2002).

Before we can begin to acquire the necessary skills, we need to examine what it means to nurse a multiethnic population. A useful starting point is to examine the language used in the literature about 'transcultural' nursing, as this is diverse and can lead to confusion for care providers and patients/ clients if used inappropriately. In this chapter, we look at some of the key concepts that underpin the development of transcultural nursing, including 'race', ethnicity, ethnic minority, racism, and culture. We consider the concept of human rights and how the Human Rights Act 1998 underpins policy-making in multiethnic Britain. Models of transcultural care are examined as frameworks for providing culturally competent assessments for patients/clients requiring health-care interventions.

Aims of transcultural nursing

Transcultural nursing is theory and practice, focused specifically on comparing the care needs of people with differences and similarities in beliefs, values, and cultures in order to provide culturally congruent, meaningful, and beneficial health care (Leininger, 1995). In understanding this definition it is important to note that transcultural nursing is an essential area of study for nurses as it enables the nurse to acquire the knowledge and skills necessary to function in a society that includes groups of people from designated cultures. The knowledge and the skills gained through such study will ensure that nurses meet the specific needs of people from different ethnic origins, thus ensuring that their care is therapeutic and meaningful. People from different backgrounds will quickly become distrustful, discontented and unhappy with their care if nurses show little knowledge or skill in meeting their particular health-care needs. In order to begin to acquire the knowledge and skills needed nurses should gain an understanding of the particular cultures that form part of the society or population they are caring for, including the beliefs, the values, lifestyles and religious practices engaged in.

Nurses who are skilled in transcultural nursing believe it is the human right of every culture to have their beliefs, values and practices understood and respected by those providing care. This means that this particular area of study is as important to nurses as studying anatomy and physiology, biology, ethics and nursing practice. Indeed many of these areas are experienced in different ways by people of different cultures. For example, the dietary habits of a particular cultural group will affect the nursing practice of assisting someone to eat and drink. Similarly, the native language of a particular group of people will affect the way in which the nurse communicates with individual people on a range of health-care issues.

The goal of transcultural nursing is to prepare nurses who are culturally competent, knowledgeable, sensitive and safe to practice in a multicultural environment. Achievement of this goal must begin with the development of an awareness of one's own ethnic identity, as this enables longstanding biases, misunderstandings and prejudices to be expelled, which may otherwise make it difficult for nurses to become culturally competent. So, before we can examine what it means to nurse a multiethnic population, we need to know something about the concepts of race, ethnicity, ethnic minority, racism, human rights, and culture. We need to know what is meant and – just as important – what is *not* meant, by these terms.

Race

One of the most difficult concepts for nurses to come to terms with is the idea of 'race' and idea that people belong to different 'races'. In fact a wide range of biologists and population geneticists agree that there is *no scientific basis for claiming that people belong to different 'races'* (Rose *et al*, 1984; Cavilli-Sforza *et al*, 1996). The word 'race' is therefore placed in inverted commas to show that, although the term is used in everyday language, it has no basis in fact.

Culley and Dyson (2001) discuss the problems inherent within the language used to define and describe people from different cultural groups. They begin by commenting on the notion that there are groups of people so biologically distinct that they form separate racial groups or races. They argue that this notion has been scientifically discredited as there is a great deal of genetic variation within so-called 'races' and a great deal of genetic overlap between them. Therefore terms such as 'Caucasian' for example, which is often used as part of a scheme of racial classification, is inappropriate as it carries connotations of biological race. Culley and Dyson (2001) suggest that the very idea of biological races has been associated with much malevolence and hatred, and dates back to a time when Britain had a colonial empire and the classification of 'races' was based on a notion of a hierarchy of 'races' (that some races were allegedly superior to others). They go on to suggest that an alternative to the term 'race' is the term 'ethnicity' because this is used to socially construct differences grounded in culture, ancestry and language rather than in supposed physical or biological differences. Culley and Dyson note that 'race' (2001) – even though it has no significant scientific basis – is still used frequently as people persist with the view that there are distinct racial groups (look at the work of the Commission for Racial Equality at http://www.cre.gov.uk/).

You may have also heard the word 'black' used frequently to describe people from minority ethnic groups. However, while you may think this is acceptable to both the patient/client and the professional or lay health-care worker, because it is used so frequently in discussions of 'race' and health, it is not clearly defined and often used without any clear understanding of the collectivities being referred to (Sheldon and Parker, 1992). For example, 'black' is sometimes used to refer to all minority ethnic groups and sometimes to African and African–Caribbean groups. This can lead to confusing and potentially misleading accounts, as Culley and Dyson (2001) point out. Similarly, in a health-care situation, for example, when admitting someone into hospital and undertaking an initial assessment, a nurse may choose to describe them as 'black' when identifying their ethnic origin. This may occur because the nurse makes the assumption that all minority ethnic groups refer to themselves in that way. However, this assumption can be challenged in that while many Caribbean's use the term 'black' as a form of self-identity, people from the Indian sub-continent may not readily define themselves in that way (Modood, 1998). Additionally the notion of a collective political identity, shared by those who experience racism and exclusion by the 'white' majority in Britain, continues to underpin the practice of self-defined Black organisations in Britain: as For example, The 1990 Trust or Operation Black Vote. Quite simply, you must be careful about the use of the term 'black' by yourself or others as it currently enjoys no unambiguous consensual usage.

The term 'white' is also problematic, often being employed interchangeably with English, British and European. This leads to confusion between notions of nationality or citizenship with concepts of ethnicity. In the context of health care, it is clear that there are 'white' minority groups, whose needs are often overlooked, including, for example, Irish, Polish, Bosnian, and Serbian groups. There has, in recent years, been a significant amount of academic literature that has sought to explore the nature and social construction of 'whiteness' in Western European cultures (see for example, Dyer, 1997; Kincheloe *et al*, 1998; Hage, 1998).

The terms 'black' and 'white' are ambiguous and have political implications whereby classifying people into either Black or White has shown a tendency to assume that society can be divided into an oppressed Black minority and a dominant White majority (Culley and Dyson, 2001). This has lead to the use of other terms by nurses in an effort to avoid causing offence. One such word is 'coloured', while another is to refer to someone as an 'immigrant'. Both of these words are problematic. For example, in South Africa during the period of Apartheid, the term 'coloured' was used as part of the classification of 'races' by the State in effecting systematic discrimination. Therefore 'coloured' may be offensive to some people. A nurse who unthinkingly refers to an individual as 'coloured' when that person has experienced racial discrimination by being classified on the basis of 'colour', may cause anxiety and resentment. The nurse may also become the target of abuse from anyone who does not describe him- or herself (or want to be described) as 'coloured'. Similarly, to refer to all members of ethnic groups as 'immigrant' is inappropriate because, while it may apply and be acceptable to some older members, the majority of the members of that group will have been born in the UK (Culley and Dyson, 2001).

Ethnicity

As an alternative to the discredited notion of so-called distinct biological races, social scientists refer to 'ethnicity'. Ethnicity is a difficult term to define, but most commentators agree that it refers to people who share a common ancestry and who perhaps can trace this ancestry to a shared geographical area of the world (Bradby, 1995). Such peoples may also (but not necessarily) share language, religion, diet, dress, and social customs. As such, the term 'ethnicity' refers to *everybody*, for all these characteristics apply equally to 'White English' people and all 'other' peoples. It would therefore be inaccurate (and indeed nonsensical) to refer to an 'ethnic' diet, an 'ethnic' style of dress or home decoration, or indeed to 'ethnic' health.

The concept of ethnicity is not without its problems especially as it is used in nursing and by nurses. There is no single, universally accepted concept of ethnicity and this in itself poses problems for nurses caring for people from diverse multiethnic groups. One such problem is identified by Serrant-Green (2001) who describes herself as a Black nurse lecturer and writes of the problem of referring to individuals from minority ethnic groups as 'other'. While Serrant-Green wrote predominantly about nurses from minority ethnic groups, her argument is relevant for nurses of any ethnic background (we all have an 'ethnicity'). She discusses the tendency, in attempting to learn about the cultures, values, attitudes and beliefs of patients/clients in an effort to become 'culturally-sensitive, to see them as belonging to a minority ethnic group and viewed as 'other' or 'different to' the professional. Serrant-Green suggests that this phenomenon instead of promoting transcultural nursing in fact contradicts any attempt to value diversity by denying the existence of the minority ethnic nurse. Her view applies equally to all nurses of all ethnic groups, for as Culley and Dyson (2001) point out ethnicity is something we all have. To talk about 'ethnic diet', 'ethnic dress' or 'my ethnic clients' is to talk about 'all diets', 'all dress codes' and 'all clients'. Nurses who have the knowledge and skills to engage in transcultural nursing care should recognise that we are all 'ethnic', yet our ethnicity does not define us. We all need our identity to be respected, yet we cannot be adequately understood in terms of our ethnicity as it is overlaid by gender, age, socio-economic and professional identities (Gerrish *et al*, 1996a). These factors may be more or less significant in any specific context or at any specific point in time. For example, the nurse caring for someone who is experiencing pain (who as part of their culture does not accept analgesia) would need to recognise and respect this, while having an understanding of what is acceptable to them, in order to meet their health-care needs. Leininger and McFarland (2002) refer to this as 'holding' knowledge and suggest it helps nurses respond appropriately to cultural pain differences in therapeutic and sensitive ways and to *not* assume that everyone experiences physical, emotional and cultural pain in the same way. This is the essence of transcultural nursing.

It has been noted that some confusion surrounds the terms 'ethnicity' and 'nationality' (Culley and Dyson, 2001). 'Nationality' refers to the nation state in which you have citizenship (British, for example), or your country of or place of birth (for example, England, Scotland, Wales, Ireland, India,

Pakistan, Kenya, Uganda, Zimbabwe, Jamaica, or Bosnia). On the other hand 'ethnicity' refers to peoples with a common ancestry, and is usually linked to a particular geographical territory, perhaps sharing a common language, religion or other social customs. Ethnic identity is concerned with the way in which people define themselves and their relationships to others (Mason, 1995). Nurses may find themselves in a position of caring for patients/clients from a variety of different ethnic backgrounds, depending on the prevalence of that particular group in the community. This requires the nurse to have an understanding of the knowledge and skills that are prerequisites for effective transcultural nursing, for example, procedures for contacting interpretation services, for meeting dietary needs, or for caring for people of different faiths throughout the process of death and dying. Look at The Local Interfaith Guide at http://www.interfaith.org.uk/.

We can see that to use the term 'ethnicity' is not without its problems for some nurses. Not least, as already noted, it may encourage those nurses who, while attempting to acquire the knowledge and skills to care effectively for people from multicultural backgrounds, come to view those being cared for as 'other' than themselves. This has led to some groups in society being referred to as belonging to an ethnic minority. According to the Runnymede Trust (2000): "The term 'minority' has connotations of 'less important' or 'marginal'. In many settings it is not only insulting but also mathematically misleading or inaccurate. Further, its use perpetuates the myth of white [*sic*] homogeneity – the notion that everyone who does not belong to a minority is by that token a member of a majority in which there are no significant differences or tensions".

There is more to read on this issue at http://www.runnymedetrust.org/. It is important for nurses to ensure that whatever the social customs that characterise the ethnic group being cared for, these customs are not ignored, but respected and facilitated. These customs may include dietary practices, religious practices, dress, social interactions within groups, or specific rituals engaged in during periods of ill health, death and dying.

Most communities are now considered to be 'multiethnic' due to significant changes in world demography during the last century, and this presents considerable challenges for those involved in all aspects of health-care provision (Papadopoulos and Lees, 2002). Nurses need to be responsive to the different needs, experiences, values and beliefs of ethnically diverse populations. This requires nurses to gain an understanding of their own ethnic identity in order to recognise and respect the ethnic identity of the person being cared for.

Ethnic minority

The expression 'ethnic minority' usually means an ethnic group that is in the minority *numerically* speaking, and that it is less powerful economically or politically than the ethnic majority groups. Consider the Runnymede Trust's comments about the term 'minority' (above). While the term 'minority ethnic group' is quite widely used, it is important to remember several things in interpreting its use.

- There are instances where the numerically smaller ethnic groups are politically and economically dominated by the numerically larger ethnic group. For example, in the UK those who self-describe as 'White British' are in the majority numerically but also enjoy better material living conditions and better health status than, say, those of Pakistani Muslim descent (Nazroo, 1997).
- There are instances where the numerically smaller group is the politically and economically more powerful group (for example, in South Africa during the Apartheid era the Black population were numerically in the majority but were politically and economically oppressed).
- Within the ethnic group who self-describe as 'White British', there are many significant ethnic differences – differences that are often not thought about. As we have seen, someone who self-describes as 'White English' might derive their ancestry from first century Romans, tenth century Vikings, eleventh century Normans, eighth century French Huguenots, nineteenth century Ashkenazi Jews or Irish, or from twentieth century Italian or Polish emigrants (to give just a few examples).
- Within the group who self-describe as 'White British', there are also significant differences other than ethnicity. How people respond to and 'live' within a particular society will vary according to their socio-economic status, their gender, their age, their religion. Think about disaggregating the idea of homogenous (that is, all the same) ethnic groups. There are significant differences within both 'White' and minority ethnic groups. We all need our ethnic identity to be respected, but we cannot be understood just in terms of our ethnicity.
- There are increasing numbers of people who may identify with more than one ethnic group. For example, a person may have a father of Black British (Caribbean) descent and a mother of 'White British' descent. While some may wish to assert their identity as 'Black' and others their identity as 'White' many will wish to recognise their dual

heritage. At the moment we do not even have concepts for recognising and respecting these identities, except through inaccurate and clumsy terms such as 'mixed race'.

Ethnic monitoring

One of the activities that a modern nurse is required to undertake as part of professional record-keeping is 'ethnic monitoring'. At the time of writing the Department of Health requires that this be carried out using ethnic categories devised for the UK 2001 Census (see *Appendix*). However, ethnic monitoring is not just collecting ethnic data on individuals who use the health services. 'Ethnic recording' is the actual task of asking the patient/client to complete a form to indicate their ethnic origin (Johnson, 2001). Ethnic monitoring suggests a number of other features. These include:

- A commitment to maintain these records over time and not just as an isolated initiative.
- A commitment to explain to the patient/client the reason for the data collection.
- A commitment to monitor the patterns in the data to see if they reveal any possible inequities or unintended or deliberate discrimination.
- A commitment to tackle any discrimination revealed by monitoring such patterns.
- A commitment to use such data for planning appropriate services in the future.

One of the reasons for ethnic monitoring is to see if there is racial discrimination in service provision and/or in the manner in which services are provided. Although there is no scientific basis to the term 'race', it is a concept that has been used as a powerful and damaging concept in effecting discrimination against certain peoples (Henley and Schott, 1999). In other words, while there is no reality to 'race' there is a reality to 'racism'.

Racism

'Racism' can be defined as a combination of ideas and practices, based on the false assumption that there are separate and distinct human races. These ideas and practices are then used to socially exclude peoples on the basis of the false belief that they belong to these distinct 'racial' groups. 'Racial prejudice' is the holding of attitudes, while 'racism' refers to actions that put such prejudice into effect. Racism can take many forms as described here.

Physical violence

In the late-twentieth century a number of cities established racial attacks monitoring projects in order to establish both the reality and the extent of physical attacks against minority ethnic communities.

Racialism

An example of this is name-calling.

Direct racial discrimination

This is when the racial prejudice that a person has is deliberately acted upon with intent to harm the person physically, mentally or socially. For example, a patient refusing attempts to care for them, or a White worker refusing to sit next to a Black colleague or to work for them, or White and Black colleagues refusing to engage in exchange of everyday pleasantries.

Indirect racial discrimination

Examples include having to take additional entrance tests, disproportionately not receiving official rewards, or being refused choices in work patterns afforded to others.

Racial stereotyping

There are numerous instances in the health literature of staff and/or patients/ clients stereotyping minority ethnic peoples in various ways. Some of the myths and false notions a practising nurse must avoid are: (1) that African or Caribbean people are as always happy-go-lucky; have magical powers of healing; or are knowledgeable about tropical diseases (see Culley *et al*, 2001); (2) that women of Pakistani Muslim descent are rude, quick in child-birth and 'keep themselves to themselves' (see Bowler, 1993); (3) that various peoples of Indian, Pakistani or Bangladeshi descent 'look after their own' in extended families and therefore do not need formal social-care services (Atkin and Rollings, 1996); (4) that Black and Asian people have different pain thresholds from White people or that Black people may exaggerate their pain in order to get the drugs they want (see Anionwu and Atkin, 2001).

Racialising health differences

Much racism is based on skin colour, but some groups are subjected to what has been called cultural or 'new racism', whereby the target is not a racially defined group but one regarded as *culturally* distinct. An example of this is the discrimination and prejudice shown towards some South Asian Muslim people in the UK, and the manner in which various cultural practices, such as consanguineous marriage, have come to be regarded by health professionals as 'problems'(Ahmad, 2000).

Institutional racism

Racism can be defined as the actions of a prejudiced individual who may act in a derogatory or discriminatory way towards another individual or group. This is sometimes called personal or individual racism. However, racism can also be 'institutional'. This kind of racism was highlighted in the 1999 *Macpherson Report* (Macpherson, 1999), an inquiry into the racist murder, in 1993, of the Black teenager Stephen Lawrence. In this case, there may not have been any intention to discriminate on the part of individuals, but the effect of doing things in customary ways and not taking account of diversity can result in a discriminatory outcome. In this case, racism is indirect and embedded in the institution itself. Other examples include failing to provide an interpreter when needed, or failure to provide culturally appropriate food, or insisting that all nurses wear a uniform that reveals their legs.

'Institutional racism' occurs when the policies, procedures and practices of institutions have the consequence of producing, intentionally or not, outcomes that are discriminatory and that continue the cycle of disadvantage. The term gained wider currency as a concept in everyday use following the 1999 *Macpherson Report*.

The Race Relations (Amendment) Act 2000 places an onus on public bodies in Britain, to develop 'race equality schemes', and should provide health trusts in the UK with the impetus to overcome institutional racism by developing robust anti-racist policies. Under such Race Equality Schemes, public authorities will have to:

1. Assess whether their functions and policies are relevant to race equality.
2. Monitor their policies to see how they affect race equality.
3. Assess and consult on policies they are proposing to introduce.
4. Publish the results of their consultations, monitoring and assessments.
5. Ensure the public have access to the information and services they provide.
6. Train their staff on the new duties.

Human rights

Human rights are important to everyone living in Britain today. All citizens of Britain are entitled to have their basic human rights respected, but, equally, they must respect the rights of others. Human rights are those rights described as the most basic and fundamental values on which a society has been built, in other words, the rights we all take for granted. Such as:

- The right to life.
- The right to freely express one's views.
- The right to respect for one's private and family life.

Human rights have relevance in many areas of daily life, including receipt of health care. Human rights apply equally to everyone, irrespective of race, colour, religion, or culture. We have rights because we are entitled to them as human beings, regardless of personal circumstances, beliefs, religion or culture. Human rights are therefore something on which we can all find common ground – we should all be able to believe in, rely upon and exercise our rights and responsibilities.

The European Convention on Human Rights (ECHR), as well as several United Nations (UN) conventions and other international instruments exist to recognise and reinforce basic human rights and to provide a framework within which governments must act. The ECHR has been in existence since the 1950s, but has been given further force in the UK through the Human Rights Act 1998. Under the Human Rights Act, all public authorities in the UK, including health authorities, must act in accordance with the Convention rights in everything they do.

These Acts provide a framework within which Ministers, the Parliament and public authorities must operate in conducting their activities, the aim of which is to ensure that human rights are properly protected and that we are able to claim the protection of the 'Convention rights' in our own national courts. The following Articles within the framework are particularly appropriate to ensuring equality of human rights within health-care provision, whether in the acute or community setting:

Article 9 Human Rights Act: Freedom of thought, conscience and religion

Everyone has the right to freedom of thought, conscience and religion; this right includes freedom to change his religion or belief and freedom, either alone or in community with others and in public or private, to manifest his religion or belief, in worship, teaching, practice and observance.

Freedom to manifest one's religion or beliefs shall be subject only to such limitations as are prescribed by law and are necessary in a democratic society in the interests of public safety, for the protection of public order, health or morals, or the protection of the rights and freedoms of others.

Article 14 Human Rights Act: Prohibition of discrimination

The enjoyment of the rights and freedoms set forth in this convention shall be secured without discrimination on any ground such as sex, race, colour, language, political or other opinion, national or social origin, association with a national minority, property, birth or other status.

The Human Rights Act 1998 provides a framework for ensuring that all members of the UK's increasingly diverse population are appropriately considered by those formulating policy and by those putting policy into effect, in this case health care policy. For a full and detailed explanation of the Human Rights Act 1998 see http://www.dca.gov.uk/peoples-rights/human-rights/.

Culture

Culture is a wider concept than ethnicity. We also need to bear in mind that culture is constantly changing and evolving and is not a fixed property of individuals. We do behave according to cultural norms (what we eat, how we interact and so on) but they are flexible guidelines rather than rules that rigidly determine human behaviour. Thinking about culture in this way helps avoid stereotyping people.

Attempts to incorporate a consideration of culture into nursing have been problematic (Ahmad, 1996), namely because of the following factors:

- There is an assumption that culture is the cause of a health problem. For example, the 1970s 'Stop Rickets' campaign assumed that the vitamin D deficiency suffered by British Asian people was culturally based, associated with not getting enough sunlight because of not going outside, when in reality it was because their staple foods, like chapati flour or rice, were not fortified with vitamin D (as is the case, by law, with margarine).
- There is an assumption that it is culture, rather than socio-economic circumstance, that is the cause of ill-health. Thus British Indian people have been accused of having poor heart health because of the use of ghee for cooking, when in fact their self-reported heart health is as good, if not better, than that of White people (Nazroo, 1999). The occurrence of birth defects in British Pakistani Muslim babies has been unfairly and judgementally linked to the practice of encouraging first-cousin (consanguineous) marriages. Ahmad (1994) commented that the research studies which suggested a relationship between cultural practice and birth disabilities were flawed because they did not account for the levels of material poverty disproportionately suffered by those same communities – which might explain the observed difference. Furthermore, consanguineous marriages are not practiced by all British Pakistani Muslim communities.
- There is an assumption that everyone within a culture will have the same social location for their experiences. We might learn that Pakistani women 'do the month' whereby they withdraw from public life for a month after giving birth to be cared for by female relatives. However, Ahmad points out this is not the experience of wealthy urban Pakistani women who might choose a high-tech elective caesarean, nor rural poor women whose material needs may mean a return to physical labour almost immediately after giving birth.
- There is failure to see that culture can be nurturing and supportive of health.

Note, then, that we follow, or adapt or even ignore our social customs, depending upon particular circumstances.

- **Not everyone in the group does it** – for example, some will not drink tea because they prefer coffee, or because they do not drink anything with caffeine in it because they regard caffeine as a drug.
- **They may do it but not all the time** – for example, some may only

attend church for special occasions, such as christenings and weddings, or at special times of year, such as carol services at Christmas, or at times of family crisis, such as the illness of a loved one.

- **They may hold to a belief underlying the activity but not be active** – there are many who regard themselves as believing in the Christian God (72% according to the UK 2001 Census), but who never go to church to express their beliefs formally.
- **They may actively reject one or more aspects of these customs** – a number may be vegetarians and so not eat fish; others may not believe in a god.
- **They may be reluctant participants in an activity** – some people may not drink alcohol and may not like the atmosphere and culture of pubs, but may go there because it they are major venues for a gathering of their friends.
- **They may change over time, or be inconsistent in beliefs** – such change may be evident in a person with over twenty years' experience in nursing, for example in the way that nurses are taught to respond to death, pain and distress in patients/clients and relatives.
- **Being ill, or being in hospital may itself change what people want** – someone may change their eating and drinking habits because they want to cheer themselves up or treat themselves because they are ill or in unfamiliar surroundings.

As the above discussion shows, an understanding of the concepts underpinning transcultural care is an important prerequisite for nurses caring for anyone in multicultural Britain. We have considered key concepts including race, ethnicity, ethnic minority, ethnic monitoring, racism, human rights and culture as important to our understanding of the experience of people from multiethnic groups in receipt of health care. In order to apply theory to practice we now move on to consider a number of models of transcultural care that have been formulated by experts in the field. The choice of model is a personal and professional one and dictated by factors including the client group, the health care setting and the philosophy of care. The aim here is to provide an overview of models of transcultural care that can aid nurses in the integration of the theory and practice of transcultural care, and not a definitive guide. The Intercultural Sensitivity model (Bennett, 1986), the Transcultural Nursing Assessment model (Giger and Davidhizar, 1998), the Sunrise model (Leininger, 1995), and the Papadopoulos, Tilki and Taylor model for Developing Cultural Competence (Papadopoulos, 2006), are examples of frameworks that can be used in conjunction with the nursing process to provide culturally sensitive care for a range of client groups.

Transcultural nursing models

Cultural competency is the ability to care for people in a culturally sensitive and appropriate manner. The development of respect for others is vital for the improvement of cultural competency. Many models explain how cultural beliefs evolve and progress and we need to examine these to see how they fit with our own cultural development.

The Intercultural Sensitivity model

Bennett's model (Bennett, 1986) attempts to explain cultural development as a continuum with six distinct stages that an individual or society can be guided through. The stages of the model are described below:

Denial of cultural differences

Individuals at this initial stage appear unaware that cultural differences exist within society – they are in denial. The aim, at this stage, is to promote recognition of the presence of diverse cultural differences within the individual's environment.

Defence of one's own culture

Bennett's second stage suggests that cultural difference is not perceived. During the first stage the individual is unable to see cultural difference, but once awareness is there the individual may feel threatened. 'Defence' arises when the individual is only able to perceive their own cultural existence as the norm; anything outside of this is viewed negatively. The aim during this second stage is to promote the similarities between different cultures, and to recognise and appreciate the differences.

Minimisation of other cultures in order to protect one's own cultural identity

Although differences are now perceived, in language and culture, the individual has still to recognise that one's own values and beliefs are part of their own ethnicity; there is still a tendency to project one's own culture onto others. At this stage, Bennett suggests that it is necessary for the individual to learn more about their own culture, in order to place it into the context of society.

Cultural acceptance

The fourth stage of Bennett's model suggests that the individual will be able to accept cultural differences once a shift in perspective is achieved. This change in perspective is accompanied by an awareness and understanding of the different meanings of behaviour across diverse cultures.

Adaptation to cultural differences

The individual should now be able to operate successfully within another culture. Bennett informs us that the development at this stage involves two steps: 'cognitive adaptation' and 'behavioural adaptation'. This is where the individual has sufficient knowledge of their own and another culture, and where they are able to assess and evaluate behaviour to the appropriate norms of the second culture.

Integration of full cultural awareness into everyday interactions

During this stage the individual is able to move between different cultures competently; they are able to draw on their knowledge of different cultural perspectives and frameworks.

There has been some debate about the value of looking at culture as a way of understanding aspects of health, for example, the differences in the health status of ethnic groups. Some writers claim that in focusing on aspects of culture the real issues that effect health status are given little attention, for example, differences in socio-economic status and/or racism (Smaje, 1996; Culley, 2001). However, Bennett's model does at least provide a framework for examining our own attitudes towards our culture, how we came to understand our culture, and how this fits in with our thinking about other cultures. Where each individual nurse lies on the continuum depends on their life experiences, and the overall aim of the model is to move the nurse towards higher levels of cultural competency through the presentation of specific content and exposure to different cultural experiences.

The Transcultural Nursing Assessment model

Giger and Davidhizar (1998) developed a model for assessing differences between people in various cultural groups. The model can be used to guide curriculum content where the intention is to facilitate competency in transcultural nursing or to facilitate a transcultural nursing assessment of patients and clients. Giger and Davidhizar's model has similar aims to those enshrined within Bennett's Intercultural Sensitivity model, that is to facilitate culturally safe practice. However, this model considers six additional interrelated factors:

- Communication
- Space
- Social organisation
- Time
- Environmental control
- Biological variations.

Giger and Davidhizar explain that understanding these concepts provides a first step towards appreciating the diversity that exists between people from varied backgrounds. It should be noted that Giger and Davidhizar do not claim that all persons reflect, in full or in part, their cultural or ethnic group of origin, rather ethnicity and cultural identity are derived from and are influenced by a variety of factors including socialisation, socio-economic status, political factors, and environment. Culture may shift as people move within and between other groups in society for as Ahmad (1996) points out culture is dynamic and contextual, not rigid and unchanging. Similarly, ethnicity may also be affected by contextual factors with diversity present within some ethnic groups. Consider, for example, a number of generations of a Muslim family living in Great Britain where the older members were born in India or Pakistan with the younger members born in the UK. There may be quite varied expressions of ethnicity within this family, derived from each individual member's life experiences, socialisation, environment, political and socio-economic status.

Communication

Communication is seen to provide the means by which people connect. It is seen as a continuous process by which one person interacts with another through written or oral language, gestures, facial expressions, and body language. The authors believe that communication and culture are closely intertwined; furthermore communication is the means by which culture is transmitted and preserved. Culture influences how feelings are expressed and the type of verbal and non-verbal expressions that are appropriate. In the context of health care, cultural influences on communication are important when making an initial assessment and in subsequent assessments if inappropriate decisions regarding care are to be avoided. The communication practices of each cultural group affect the expression of ideas and feelings, decision-making and communication strategies that nurses can draw on in order to provide transculturally competent care. A person's communication reflects, determines, and consequently moulds the culture. On the other hand, a culture may be limited and moulded by its communication practices (Giger and Davidhizar, 1998). As people age, they consolidate their own communicative style, which may become a powerful expression of their identity and life experience. Language and modes of expression do not remain static within cultures and all of us may find generational shifts in patterns of communication that make age an increasingly significant factor in our experience of communicating. Of course, for some, memory loss and changes in personal priorities and interest also change their capacity to interact (see *Chapter Six*). There are changes that may be anticipated irrespective of ethnic identity.

Space

'Personal space is the area that surrounds a person's body; it includes both the space and the objects within that space. Personal space is seen to be an extension of the body and is also referred to as 'outer' space, with 'inner' space referring to the personal state of consciousness or awareness. Davidhizar and Giger (1998) propose that a person's comfort level is related to personal space; discomfort is experienced when personal space is invaded. Although personal space is an individual matter and varies with the situation, the dimensions of the 'comfort zone' also vary from culture to culture. Ethnic groups frequently differ in their need for space. For example, some Black African people may relate to others with closer proximity than, for example, some Asian people. The transculturally competent nurse will recognise that different people have differing spatial needs, as illustrated, for example, when conversing with others, or when resting and/or recuperating.

Social organisation

Cultural behaviour, or how a person acts in a given situation is dependent on the process of socialisation. Socialisation involves the acquisition of knowledge and the internalisation of values. One's own cultural competency is achieved through the process of socialisation, when, for example, as children we watch adults' behaviour in certain ways and we infer certain rules of behaviour. Giger and Davidhizar (1998) propose that patterns of cultural behaviour are important to the nurse because they provide explanations for behaviour related to life events, for example, birth, death, puberty, childbearing, illness and disease. As children we learn certain beliefs about these life events and the learned behaviours generally persist throughout life, ensuring that we act in certain ways in the event of similar experiences. The transculturally competent nurse needs not only to be sensitive to how this dimension of social organisation has implications for their understanding of their patient/clients' needs; but also (and equally importantly) needs to sustain a reflexive awareness of how the social organisation of their working environment impacts upon their consciousness and routine practice.

Time

Time is considered to be one of humanity's greatest mysteries (Giger and Davidhizar, 1998). As such, it is through the awareness and conception of time that the products of the human mind seem to possess an existence apart from the passage of time, which is seen to be a personal perception. While the concept of time may be familiar to most people regardless of cultural heritage, the development of an awareness of time is neither simple nor universally the same. Perception of time depends on culture and may be concrete or abstract, something that can be controlled, or over which people have no control. In a similar way, temporal orientation (ordering of the past, present and future) may differ between and within cultures. For example, some people will be satisfied to know that they will be undergoing a particular medical test in the future, while others will need more precise information about times and dates. For the nurse, it is necessary to understand how time is perceived within different cultures in order to communicate appropriately and effectively with people. For example, if the nurse informs the patient or client that a surgical procedure is to be carried out the following day and therefore is required to abstain from eating and drinking, but fails to explain when this is to commence and why it is necessary, then that individual may refrain from eating and drinking immediately or may ignore the need to do so at the designated time.

Environmental control

Environmental control relates to the individual's perception of their ability to direct or influence factors in the environment. This view incorporates the idea that the 'environment is more than just the place where someone lives or where care or treatment occurs. The term 'environment' encompasses all the systems and processes that affect each individual. On a practical level, for nurses engaged in transcultural care it is important to understand the views of the patient or client regarding their ability to control their environment. For example, some cultures have a fatalistic view, tending to accept the status quo without the need for rational explanation. They are more likely to accept diagnosis and prognosis without the need for further clarification, treatment options, and alternative or complementary therapies. In contrast, other cultures value the ability to be in control, to dominate and to explain/have explanations for their environmental circumstances. It is incumbent on nurses endeavouring to provide culturally appropriate care to understand what is required by each individual in terms of explanations, likely outcomes, and to respect this aspect of culture as it manifests itself. And as already noted the transculturally competent nurse should have a reflexive understanding of the determination of their behaviour; both at the general level of their own cultural context and at the specific level of their 'community of practice'. Guaranteeing culturally safe practice may require challenging institutional routines as much as it demands the development of personal competences.

Biological variations

The Transcultural Nursing Assessment model recognises that people differ culturally according to communication, spatial relationships and needs, social organisations, time orientation and ability to describe the environment (Giger and Davidhizar, 1998). However, less well recognised and certainly far more debatable is the view that biological differences exist among people of different ethnic groups. The authors of the Transcultural Nursing Assessment model suggest that for many years biological differences between races were underplayed and remained unrecognised. They discuss a rapidly growing body of knowledge relating to these differences, referred to as 'biocultural ecology'. The authors propose that failure to recognise 'ethnic differences' with a biological basis may lead to more racism or ethnocentrism than if these differences are ignored. Assessment of the patient/client for biocultural factors that impact on health is an essential component of culturally sensitive care. Contrary to this Rose *et al*, (1984) suggest that there is no scientific basis for the notion of distinct 'racial' groups. Furthermore, there is potentially more genetic variation between two Black people than between either one of those two Black people and a White person. This is because only a fraction of inherited characteristics are visible (such as skin colour). Rose *et al*, (1984) argue that the division of the human species into 'races' on the basis of the incidence of certain types of gene frequencies reflect social decisions, not an underlying biological classification. Dyson and Smaje (2001) point out that a distinction needs to be drawn between arguing for a biological basis to 'racial groups' (which they reject) and the argument that there can be specific genetic factors that are broadly correlated with some socially ascribed 'ethnic' identities. They argue that there is geographical variation within the human species in genetic constitution. However, it is as a result of historical patterns of human contact that socially defined 'racial' classifications also conform to a rough geographical patterning. Dyson and Smaje (2001) acknowledge that there is an association, albeit a highly imperfect one, between social groups who have been given 'racial' labels and genetic traits. They go on to point out that rejecting notions of distinct biological 'racial groups' does not mean completely rejecting genetic factors as possible explanations of health variations between ethnic groups, adding that at the same time we need to be aware of focusing too much on conditions in which genetic factors play a large contributory part, such as sickle cell disease, at the expense of conditions that affect all ethnic groups, such as heart disease, hypertension or diabetes (Smaje, 1996).

The important point to remember for nurses engaged in transcultural nursing is that in recognising that a partial association exists between ethnic group and genetic factors, genes only have an influence in the context of other genes, the whole body, the physical environment and the social environment (Rose *et al*, 1984). When viewed in this way the Transcultural Nursing Assessment model facilitates recognition of biological/genetic factors in a non-discriminatory fashion, while giving equal consideration to the cultural factors of communication, space, social organisation, time, and environmental control.

The Sunrise model

Madeleine Leininger began work on the Sunrise model in 1955 and continued to revise it in minor ways between 1955 and 1985 in relation to the theory and multiple holistic factors that she believes could influence cultural care (Leininger, 1995). Several assumptions underpin her work and a selective number of these are detailed below in order to best describe the philosophy underpinning the model.

- Care is the essence of nursing and a distinct, dominant, central, and unifying concept.
- Culturally based care is essential for well-being, health, growth, and survival and to face 'handicaps' or death.
- Culturally based care is the most comprehensive and holistic means to know, explain and interpret, and predict nursing care phenomena and to guide nursing decisions and actions.
- Every human culture has generic (lay, folk, or indigenous) care knowledge and practices and usually professional care knowledge and practices, which vary Transculturally and individually.
- Culturally congruent and beneficial nursing care can only occur when care values, expressions, or patterns are known and used explicitly for appropriate, safe, and meaningful care.

Leininger's Sunrise model shows potential influences (not causes) that might explain care practices related to historical, cultural, social structure, world view, environmental, and other factors. As such it is a useful framework for helping to understand the needs and health requirements of patients/clients. Leininger incorporates within the model features usually embedded or related to social structure such as religion, kinship, politics, and economics. Gender, age and ethnic information are embedded in family ties and specific norms and practices. The model was developed initially as a conceptual holistic research guide aimed at enabling researchers to identify the theoretical aspects of transcultural nursing (for example, how other cultures experience pain, death and dying, bereavement and to explain the nursing practices that stem from this) and she also describes how the model may be used in nursing assessment. She describes how nurses may tease out embedded practices through careful questioning, active listening, patience, and by confirming what one sees and hears, believing that patients/clients like to tell their story and are often pleased that the nurse remains interested in their world of telling and knowing.

The Sunrise model can be used by all those engaged in transcultural care. However, nurses can use it to facilitate the assessment of the total needs of patients, clients, families, groups, cultures, and communities, and even institutions. Nurses should keep in mind the central focus of nursing, but should examine cultural factors to gather information and to interpret the information in a meaningful way.

When using the Sunrise model the nurse can begin anywhere depending on the focus of the nursing assessment. For example, if the nurse identifies an urgent need to gather information relating to religious/spiritual factors for someone admitted in the terminal stages of an illness, so as to provide appropriate and culturally relevant care, then this would be the area of the model where the nurse would begin. Ultimately, the nurse would need to assess all factors in the model to get a comprehensive and accurate assessment, and this may happen over a period of time (Leininger and McFarland, 2002).

The Sunrise model guides the nurse to assess different holistic factors that tend to influence an individuals care and health. Leininger views the major areas as being assessment of the patients/client's world view, environmental context and social structure factors. In these important areas, she includes the following:

- Cultural values, beliefs, and practices
- Religious, philosophical, or spiritual beliefs
- Economic factors
- Educational beliefs
- Technology views
- Family and social ties
- Political and legal factors.

In addition to the above, the nurse assesses the general lay and professional beliefs, practices and experiences relevant to someone's cultural interpretations or experiences of health care. In other words, the nurse needs to discover what the patient/client feels and believes about health care, their expectations, their needs, wants and desires, in respect of their treatment and experience of being cared for by others.

The Sunrise model places emphasis on the necessity of assessing ethnic orientation and the environmental context in which the patient/client finds themselves. For example, home conditions, access to particular types of food (eg. vegetarian, vegan, Halal, Kosher), or family access to transport.

The aim of the Sunrise model is to enable a comprehensive picture to be gained of the individuals daily living environment and the nurse needs to make this assessment with a health-care focus drawing on other members of the interdisciplinary team (occupational health, physiotherapist, social worker, dietician, interpreter, family support worker, family liaison worker) whenever required.

In order to ensure a comprehensive assessment and to guide you towards cultural competency in using the Sunrise model, the following guiding principles provide a suitable framework. You should:

- Show a genuine and sincere interest in the patient/client as you listen and learn from them.
- Pay attention to gender or class differences, communication needs, and interpersonal space.

- Make sure you are completely familiar with the Sunrise model, its underpinning assumptions and its use in practice before commencing the transcultural nursing assessment.
- During the assessment remain fully conscious of your own cultural orientation, biases and prejudices.
- Remain aware that some patients/clients may belong to special groups (eg. the homeless or gay/lesbian community, drug users, and the mentally ill). These groups need to be respected, and their rights understood, and heard, and assessment made in order to ensure culturally appropriate care.
- Be aware of your cultural competency or areas in need of development before using the assessment tool.
- Make sure you inform the patient/client and all significant others about the assessment, the date and time you intend to carry it out, in order to gain consent and to ensure full and complete understanding of the purpose of the transcultural assessment.
- Make sure you make a holistic assessment, by using all appropriate parts of the Sunrise model.
- Remain an active listener throughout the assessment.
- Following the assessment, reflect on the information gathered in relation to your transcultural nursing knowledge.

The model for Developing Cultural Competence

The definition of cultural competence underpinning the Papadopoulos, Tilki and Taylor model for Developing Cultural Competence is the capacity to provide effective health care, taking into consideration people's cultural beliefs, behaviours and needs (Papadopoulos, 2006). It is argued that cultural competence is both a process and an output, and results from the synthesis of knowledge and skills that are acquired during personal and professional life and are added to constantly. The resulting model of cultural competence is underpinned by a set of values based on human rights, socio-political systems, intercultural relations, human ethics and human caring. The following is an outline of the model as described by the authors.

Cultural awareness

The first stage of the model covers cultural awareness, beginning with an examination of personal values and beliefs. Values and beliefs are seen as the principles used to guide life and to make decisions and judgements regarding one's life and one's dealings with others. Personal values and beliefs are said to develop from an early age and are influenced in a variety of ways by a variety of factors, for example, family, culture and social environment. When compared with the values and beliefs of a person, whether a friend or colleague form a different background, many similarities as well as some differences will emerge. It is important to recognise the importance of both similarities and differences because these define uniqueness and individuality as well as identifying shared or common ground. Of importance to the authors within the context of cultural awareness is the understanding that, while we may not be consciously aware of personal values and beliefs, these do exist at a subconscious level and may influence our behaviour and attitude towards others (Papadopoulos, 2006). In some situations and circumstances this can lead to negative judgements about others if our long-held values and beliefs cloud our ability to view others values and beliefs as legitimate. In cases where the values and beliefs of one ethnic group are seen as superior to another, a case of ethnocentricity exists. In order to avoid ethnocentric behaviour Papadopoulos (2006) draws our attention to the need to understand our own ethnic origins as a prerequisite to understanding the ethnic origins of other people and groups.

Cultural knowledge

In this next stage of the model, the authors highlight the importance of recognising how culture influences individual lifestyles, personal identity and relationships with others within and without a particular culture in the broadest possible sense. For example, through religion, dress, diet, language, art, values, attitudes and beliefs. The authors then point to sources of cultural knowledge and draw attention to the fact that these can be derived from a wide variety of disciplines such as anthology, sociology, psychology, biology, nursing, medicine and the arts. Indeed any sources, that may help explain, in a meaningful way, any aspect of culture. It is important to draw on 'expert' knowledge in understanding aspects of a culture. However, Papadopoulos (2006) recognises the importance of allowing the culture to 'speak for itself', ie. recognising the importance of giving a voice to the people who are to be effected by the decisions of others. One way of doing this is to ensure that the central question when deciding how to care for others in a culturally sensitive manner is one of whose values are used to construct the care.

Cultural sensitivity

The third stage considers cultural sensitivity, the crucial development of appropriate interpersonal relationships with patients/clients. Papadopoulos talks here of the centrality of how the professional views the person in their care, that is, as a true partner in decision-making. If the professional does not recognise the patient/client as partner-in-care then cultural sensitivity will not be achieved. In her view, true partnerships involve trust, acceptance and respect, as well as facilitation and negotiation. Of vital importance to the development of a true partnership in care is the notion of effective communication. This is brought into sharp focus when communicating across cultural boundaries and highlights the need for greater understanding of the particular culture in order to avoid miscommunication based on misunderstanding. Papadopoulos draws on the work of Kim (1992) and Gerrish *et al*, (1996b) highlighting the need for health-care professionals to develop transcultural communicative competence. The components of transcultural communicative competence are described as cultural communicative competence (whereby the nurse learns to understand cultural values, behavioural patterns and rules for interaction in specific cultures) and intercultural communication (which is the generic ability to recognise the challenges of communication across cultural boundaries).

Cultural competence

This is the final stage of the model. Cultural competence requires the synthesis and application of previously gained awareness, knowledge and sensitivity. Practical skills are recognised as important, for example, assessment of need, clinical diagnosis, and other caring skills (Papadopoulos, 2006). In this stage of the model attention is drawn to the importance of recognising and challenges racism and other forms of discriminatory and oppressive behaviour. Interestingly, Papadopoulos points to the usefulness of drawing on other writers in the field of transcultural nursing care in order to develop a comprehensive understanding of the tools available to collect cultural data, including the Sunrise model (Leininger, 1995) described earlier in this chapter. Purnell's model of Cultural Competence (Purnell and Paulanka, 1998), and Berlin and Fowkes' LEARN model (Berlin and Fowkes, 1983) for conducting a cultural assessment. The Royal College of Nursing website also provides a useful resource regarding transcultural nursing care (http://www.rcn.org.uk/resources/transcultural/).

The ever-increasing population of culturally and ethnically diverse patients/clients requires nurses to be culturally competent and sensitive.

As student nurses in the UK spend 50% of their time learning in clinical settings, recognition of distinct cultural beliefs, customs and values is essential to providing appropriate care (Gerrish, 1997). Acquisition of the knowledge and skills needed to provide culturally appropriate care depends on an in-depth understanding of the theory and practice of transcultural nursing (Leininger, 1995).

Conclusions

In conclusion, this chapter has considered the theoretical underpinnings of transcultural nursing, including the concepts of race, ethnicity, ethnic minority, racism, human rights, and culture. The importance of exploring our own ethnicity as a basis for understanding and respecting the ethnicity of others has been noted. In so doing emphasis is placed on the importance of valuing diversity without coming to view people whose cultural orientation is different to our own as 'other than' or 'apart' from ourselves. We have considered what is meant by cultural competency by looking at a number of transcultural nursing models, including Bennett's Intercultural Sensitivity model (1986), Giger and Davidhizar's Transcultural Nursing Assessment model (1998), Leininger's Sunrise model (1995), and the Papadopoulos, Tilki and Taylor model for Developing Cultural Competence as described by Papadopoulos (2006). Aspects of culture are acknowledged by giving attention to and recognising the benefit of using models of transcultural care in everyday practice, which involves people from a wide variety of cultural backgrounds. Acknowledgement is also given to the fact that, while a number of such models exist and can provide a useful framework for assessing the needs of patients/clients with specific ethnic needs, they do not replace the need for nursing knowledge in respect of the kinds of people likely to be encountered in any given area of health-care practice.

The following chapters explain how nurses can provide culturally sensitive and culturally competent care, beginning with the care of adults. Subsequent chapters then consider the care of children, people with mental health problems, and people with learning disabilities. A case-study approach is taken within each chapter to show how the assessment of culturally sensitive care should be underpinned by knowledge of the cultural context and knowledge of the physical or psychological condition of the patients/clients.

CHAPTER 3

Adult Nursing

This chapter extends understanding of how a nurse's knowledge of transcultural care can be transferred into practice in order to provide nursing care in a culturally sensitive manner. As such, it utilises the elements of the nursing process – assess, plan, implement, and evaluate – in conjunction with Roper's (Roper *et al*, 1983) Activities of Living model in a problem-solving manner – concepts that will be familiar to nurses. While it is recognised that Roper's model is predominantly focused around the physical aspects of nursing care, nonetheless its use provides a framework for describing the kinds of problems that people, in this case adults, may present with in an acute hospital setting or in the community. When combined with a transcultural nursing model the nurse is enabled to engage with the individual in a culturally sensitive manner in the provision of culturally appropriate nursing care. The chapter begins with an overview of the nursing process followed by a discussion of the Activities of Living model. Consideration is given to working with an interpreter as this is often crucial to providing culturally appropriate care.

The nursing process

The nursing process is a problem-solving framework that enables the nurse to plan care for a patient/client on an individual basis (Hogston, 2002). The nursing process is described as being cyclical, made up of four interconnecting elements, and having a dynamic nature (Pearson *et al*, 1996). It has long been a feature of nursing care in the UK and when used in conjunction with a nursing model it facilitates consistent, evidenced-based nursing care, and necessitates accurate, up-to-date care documentation. The four distinct phases (assess, plan, implement, evaluate) each have a discreet role in the nursing process, as well as being interdependent on each other. The phases are described below.

Assess

In this phase the nurse makes an assessment of the patient/client as soon as possible following admission to hospital or the first encounter in the community. The nurse uses a variety of sources to gather information about him or her, including biographical details such as name, date of birth, age, and address. Relevant medical, personal and social details are noted. The nurse may need to consult with the patient/client, or their relatives and friends, or other people of significance, in order to obtain information necessary to plan appropriate nursing care. In addition, nursing and medical notes and records, both current and previous. The records made by other health professionals who have had contact with the patient/client may also need to be consulted. The nurse makes a physical examination of the patient/client wherever possible, which enables their overall condition to be assessed. This might include, for example, an assessment of skin integrity, mobility, and breathing. The nurse will ascertain the his or her ability to perform a number of activities of living (detailed below). During the assessment phase it is usual, if the patient/client's condition allows, to obtain and record baseline observations of blood pressure, pulse, respiration, temperature and blood glucose levels, and to undertake a basic urinalysis. These observations provide a basis from which to monitor their condition, while receiving nursing and medical interventions. During the assessment phase of the nursing process, the nurse is required to draw on observational and communication skills. Observation of the patient/client provides essential information relating to skin condition, for example its colour, texture, perfusion, and hydration. Asking appropriate questions, listening carefully to the answers and accurately recording the responses are key to ensuring a patient/client-focused plan of care. Where it is not possible to consult with the patient/client, the same skills of questioning, listening and responding should be employed when communicating with significant others. The assessment phase of the nursing process can be facilitated by using a model of nursing. One such model is described in detail below. Although considered to be the starting point of the nursing process, the assessment phase is ongoing throughout the period of care.

Plan

This phase of the nursing process extends from the assessment and, in conjunction with the patient/client wherever possible, family members/carers/significant others, determines how the individuals needs, wants and desires in relation to health are to be met. There are two distinct steps in the process of planning nursing care: setting goals and identifying actions. Hogston (2002) refers to goals as a statement of what the nurse expects the patient/client to achieve (this is sometimes referred to as an objective). The person's condition dictates whether the goals are short term or long term; in many instances the goals are combination of both. The important issue is that the goals set are patient/client-centred, are realistic, achievable and measurable. Appropriate and well-written goals enable nurses to evaluate the effectiveness of the nursing interventions implemented and to make decisions regarding further planned nursing interventions.

Implement

This part of the nursing process details explicitly the care given to and received by the patient/client. It is an accurate, up-to-date account and is signed by each nurse engaged in delivering the care as detailed in the care plan. It has been described as the 'doing' phase of the nursing process, whereby the nurse delivers nursing care according to the written instructions detailed in the care plan. The nurse must ensure that accurate recording of all interventions and nursing actions takes place, in order that subsequent care can be delivered systematically and consistently by the nursing team. A well-written, accurate care plan is essential so that the evaluation phase of the nursing process can take place in a timely and appropriate fashion and meet the ongoing nursing care needs of the patient/client.

Evaluate

Evaluation takes place at designated points during the period over which the patient/client receives health care. The points of evaluation are determined by the nursing assessment which identifies the specific needs of each individual and the subsequent plan for delivering the required nursing care. Evaluation is ongoing and leads directly back to the assessment phase of the nursing process, culminating in further planning of care or discontinuation of the requirement for, or desire for, intervention.

In order to facilitate the nursing process, a number of nursing models are available that reflect certain attitudes, values, and beliefs about health, health care and nursing. When choosing a model for use in practice it should be consistent with the nursing team's attitudes, values, and beliefs about health,

health care and nursing. The model used here to describe how nursing care may be assessed, planned, implemented and evaluated is the Activities of Living model, developed by Roper *et al*, (1983). This is a well-recognised and commonly used model of nursing in the UK. However, it is important to remember that other models of nursing are available and the choice of model should be dictated by the client group for whom care is to be provided and the philosophy of nursing underpinning the nursing practice of the care providers. The Activities of Living framework incorporates a number of elements that make it applicable to adults and older people requiring care in acute and community settings. Alternative models of care might be more appropriate with other client groups, such as children, people with learning disabilities, or people with mental health problems.

The Activities of Living model

This model incorporates a life-span approach, whereby the characteristics of the person are considered with respect to prior development, current level of development, and likely future development (Safarino, 1990). In conjunction with the life-span approach an independence–dependence continuum is used. The model then incorporates a set of twelve activities of living that represent those activities engaged in by individuals whether they are sick or well. Together these elements are referred to as 'a model of living'. When using the model of living in conjunction with the nursing process, a model of nursing is utilised.

The twelve Activities Of Living (or ALs) are as follows:

- Mmaintaining a safe environment
- Breathing
- Communication
- Mobilising
- Eating and drinking
- Eliminating
- Personal cleansing and dressing
- Maintaining body temperature
- Working and playing
- Sleeping
- Expressing sexuality
- Dying.

Assessment of the patient/client is made for each activities of living, and taking into account the life-span independence–dependence continuum a plan of care is formulated. In conjunction with the nursing process and the Activities of Living framework, a model of transcultural care can be used (such as those described in the previous chapter) to ensure that a culturally sensitive care plan is developed. For example, within Giger and Davidhizar's (1998) Transcultural Nursing Assessment, each interrelated factor (communication, space, social organisation, time, environmental control, biological variations) can be used to guide an assessment within the twelve activities of living. Although it could be argued that the 'Activities of Living' model encompasses these elements, albeit in a different format, by using a combined assessment model it is envisaged that a full and complete plan of care can be formulated which takes into account all transcultural factors that affect the adult and older people from any designated ethnic group.

Undertaking an assessment of someone for whom English is not spoken or is not the preferred language requires paying attention to the means of interpretation. Successful interpersonal communication necessitates the interpretation of speech, tone and register of language, facial expressions, body language, gestures and assumptions shared between the communicants about the context of the exchange (Bradby, 2001). The distress and pain that brings people to the health service can render communication extremely difficult. Their ability to communicate in a non-native language about their cultural or religious background may be severely reduced by the nature of their illness or injury. Bradby (2001) suggests that working without a professional interpreter takes twice as much interview time as working with one. With a professional interpreter, the nurse should schedule time to establish the terms of the interview before meeting the individual and should consult him or her again once the interaction is over to confirm a common understanding of the interview. The interpreter should be given a few minutes to initiate some rapport with the patient/client prior to the nurse consultation. The nurse should try to confirm that the patient/client and interpreter speak a mutually comprehensive language and establish whether any social differences or similarities exist that might jeopardise communication (age, gender, religion) (Bradby, 2001).

Working with an interpreter

You need to consider many things when working with an interpreter.

- If possible, make time for the interpreter to discuss the aims of the encounter with the patient/client.

- Allow time for the interpreter to introduce themselves and explain their role to the patient/client and to yourself
- Allow about twice the length of time for a patient/client interview when using an interpreter. Otherwise the communication advantages you gain through the interpretation will be lost through an over-rushed consultation.
- Check that the interpreter actually speaks the patient/client's language and dialect (for example, there are several different Chinese dialects).
- Think about where the interpreter can position themselves so as best to facilitate communication. Draw how you think the nurse, interpreter and patient/client should ideally be positioned with respect to each other.
- Think about where the interpreter should position himself or herself to maintain physical privacy of the patient/client.
- Think about how the discussion should be arranged to ensure confidentiality of the encounter. Be aware that sometimes there are no equivalent words or expressions for health terms or for body parts. In many languages, for example, there are no socially acceptable words for male or female genitalia or sexual activity and interpreters will have to find other ways of explaining what they mean. They will also have to deal with their own and the patient/client's embarrassment.
- Encourage the interpreter to ask for clarification if he or she is unsure of your intended message.
- Encourage the interpreter to declare any personal views or beliefs so that all parties can be clear of the needs of the patient/client (as opposed to the nurse or the interpreter).
- Encourage the interpreter to help you understand any nuances of the patient/client's cultural context that may not be obvious to you.
- Where possible plan the interview with the patient/client in advance.
- Try to arrange professional development time with the interpreter(s) so that you can all discuss the best ways to work together.
- Think critically about the power relationship between yourself and the interpreter and the patient/client.
- Make sure that you avoid jargon, as in: 'You DNA'd last time so now we need to do a D&C or you'll end up in A&E'.
- Avoid colloquial or idiomatic expressions such as 'How would you feel in someone else's shoes?' because the concepts may not transfer to other languages or cultures.
- Prepare the interpreter for any technical information.
- Involve the interpreting team in any continuing professional education (eg. implementing the Department of Health's guidance on collection of ethnic data) or in any change of ward policy (eg. arrangements for visiting times).

In many situations you will find that an interpreter is not provided, even when the need is clear. In such cases you may have to struggle by using friends, family members and other informal, non-trained interpreters. This is not acceptable practice but sometimes it's unavoidable. You must check the relationship of the interpreter to the patient/client; take account of the level of understanding of the interpreter, and modify your language; find out if there are things that they feel unable to translate. Remember that mistranslation can cause great distress and is in fact life threatening in some circumstances. If you are using an informal interpreter, you should be very wary of the accuracy and reliability of the interview and seek to repeat it with a trained professional interpreter at the first opportunity.

Now that we have considered ways in which a transcultural assessment can be facilitated, we can begin to apply the theoretical principles learnt to practice. In the following section we will look at the transcultural care of an adult patient/client using a case-study approach, in which a man of South Asian heritage, suffering from coronary heart disease (CHD) is admitted to hospital. Knowledge of South Asian culture is considered, and is followed by a discussion of the condition itself. A nursing assessment is then described in detail, which utilises knowledge of the individual's cultural heritage and knowledge of the physical illness. In this way, culturally sensitive care can be planned and implemented which recognises not only the person's health-care needs but also the cultural context in which the experience of ill health takes place.

Case study of Mr Mohammed Khalid Qureshi

Case introduction

Mohammed Khalid Qureshi is a 71-year-old Muslim Bangladeshi gentleman, admitted to hospital via the A&E department with a history of sudden-onset chest pain. Mr Qureshi speaks very little English, usually relying on his son, who was born in Great Britain, to communicate with people outside the Bangladeshi community on his behalf. He is accompanied by his wife who speaks no English and appears to be very anxious and upset. Mohammed Khalid and his wife live with their oldest son (a businessman), and his wife and three children in a semi-detached house. Mr Qureshi's son was informed of his father's admission to hospital by his mother. However, she was unable to give him any further information. In the A&E department Mr Qureshi undergoes blood tests, x-rays

contd./..

and an electrocardiograph (ECG). He is commenced on continuous cardiac monitoring, along with continuous observations of his temperature, pulse, respiration and blood pressure. He receives analgesia for his chest pain and is transferred to the coronary care unit with a diagnosis of myocardial infarction for a period of intensive cardiac monitoring, and further investigations and treatment. He was accompanied throughout by his wife.

Background information on the cultural values, attitudes and beliefs of South Asian people

India is the largest nation in South East Asia. It was formed in 1947 with the secession of Pakistan. India is named after the river Indus, but may also be referred to as Bharat or the land of the Sage Bharata, or as Hindustan or the land of the Hindu-Kush mountain range. India is five times larger than the UK with a population of over 1 billion. In terms of beliefs, approximately 65% follow the Hindu faith, 20% follow Islam, and 12% are Sikh. There are smaller representations of other religions such as Jainism and Buddhism, and Christianity (over 40 000 Indians are Christian). The national language of India is Hindi, but other languages include Punjabi, Gujarati, Marathi, Telegu, Kannada, Malayalam, Oriya, and Assamese.

Pakistan was formed in 1947 as West and East Pakistan. East Pakistan then separated to become Bangladesh. *Pak* means 'pure' and *istan* means 'land' (hence, land of the pure). Currently the population of Pakistan is 130 million. The main faith is Islam, with approximately 97% of the population following this faith. Pakistan's main spoken language is Urdu, with other languages including Sindhi, Punjabi, and Pushtu.

Bangladesh, formerly known as East Pakistan, came into being in 1971. *Bangla* means 'Bengali' and *desh* means 'land' (land of the Bengalis). Current population figures show 122 million people currently reside in Bangladesh, the majority of whom speak Bangla, with the main religion being Islam. Most Bangladeshi people who have settled in the UK speak Syletti, which is a regional dialect. Bangladesh shares a border with India's state of West Bengal, whose people are also Bengalis.

The island of Sri Lanka, formerly known as Ceylon, gained independence in 1971. The current population is estimated at 70 million. Buddhism, Hinduism, and Islam are the main religions, and the main spoken language is Sinhalese. Tamil is spoken by Sri Lankan's in the north and east of the country, who are actively campaigning for a separate state.

People of South Asian heritage may come from a variety of backgrounds, may speak many different languages, and may practise different faiths. Migrants to Great Britain from South Asia bring with them a wealth of skills and experience. South Asian families who practice the Islamic faith follow the teachings of the *Qur'an,* and will have particular attitudes, values and beliefs that need to be understood and respected by health-care professionals. For example, in many South Asian Muslim families, aged parents usually live with their oldest son because it is considered disrespectful for old parents to live alone. According to the *Qur'an*, taking care of one's family is as important as their other religious duties (Kulwicki, 1996). However, as health-care and social-service professionals have discovered, it is a dangerous stereotype to assume that this applies in every instance. Within service provision stereotypical views about South Asian families 'looking after their own' (Ahmad and Atkin, 1996) can undermine the delivery of care.

Most Muslim men have two or three names: a *personal* name used by family members and very close friends (eg. Khalid); a *calling* name usually used by friends and acquaintances (personal and calling names may be linked together); and a *religious* name (eg. Mohammed, which is particularly sacred and should never be used alone). Some Muslim men use a hereditary name as a surname, to fit in with the British naming system (eg. Qureshi).

In some South Asian families and cultures, people are brought up to not make a fuss, to be stoical, to show strength and fortitude, and are thus regarded as 'good patients'. In other families and cultures, people are brought up to be vocal and demonstrative, traits that may include displaying agitation, moaning, crying out, rocking, chanting, calling on God, clicking their fingers or slapping themselves. The use of a pain assessment chart, such as the McGill pain questionnaire, which shows the back and front of a naked body, may be shocking and unacceptable to people who observe strict codes of modesty, or for strict Muslims for whom making images of people is forbidden (Henley and Schott, 1999). An alternative pain assessment tool, like the Faces pain assessment scale (Bieri *et al*, 1990) may be useful in such cases. However, some conservative Muslim people may be prohibited from using any tool that depicts people. The way in which each of us perceives, responds to and expresses pain is highly personal and is influenced by several factors (Melzak, 1975), including the general norms of our own society or community, as well as our childhood experiences (Henley and Schott, 1999).

Most religions and cultures contain some guidelines about purity and pollution. In South Asian culture, all body secretions including saliva, sweat, urine, faeces, vomit, blood, semen, and menstrual fluid are traditionally considered to be 'polluting'. Running water is believed to be the most effective cleansing agent. Most Muslims wash in a prescribed manner before each of the five daily prayers; it is important to them to be clean when they pray or meditate, and there may be some distress if they are unable to pray, as might happen with the presence of intravenous infusion lines. Similarly, they may feel dirty if they cannot keep clean, especially if they are bed-bound and cannot wash themselves. Being dependent on others for washing, bathing and using the toilet is humiliating for most people, regardless of background, so it is always important to protect dignity and to try to cater for their individual habits and preferences (Henley and Schott, 1999). Always washing their perineal area with running water after using the toilet is a cultural and religious requirement for Muslims, for which it is customary to use the left hand. In hospitals there should be a bidet or basin in each toilet to enable people to wash themselves with running water. Dependent people may appreciate having warm water from a jug poured over their perineal area before being taken off the commode, bedpan or toilet. As it is not possible to know who will require what assistance, it is better to offer and be refused than to have the patient/client feel uncomfortable and dirty.

Muslim men and women must perform the same religious duties, such as the five daily prayers, fasting during Ramadan, alms-giving, and pilgrimage to Mecca (Henley, 1982). They regard men and women as having the same rights, but different (though equally important) roles. In the *Qur'an* these different roles of men and women are made clear – men are responsible for all matters outside the home and for supporting their families, and women are responsible for rearing and educating children, looking after the family and running the home. Within the family, the men and women generally share decisions, with women chiefly responsible for the comfort of the family, the upbringing and moral education of the children, and the atmosphere and conduct within the home. However, in most matters outside the home woman is under the guardianship and protection of a man, whether her father, her husband, or her son if she is a widow. This may include contact with the health service (Henley, 1982). In conservative Muslim families, a rigid code of public behaviour is followed. On visits among Muslim families, men and women do not normally shake hands. They sit separately and keep their eyes down in each other's presence. Outside the family, Muslim men and women usually socialise separately. In many South Asian cultures special jewellery may be worn which symbolises good luck. Removing this jewellery is a very bad omen because it may have been worn to protect against illness and danger. In most cases there is no reason to remove such jewellery or other items of religious significance. If there is a genuine medical reason, find out the significance of the item, and wherever possible tape over it rather than remove it (Henley and Schott, 1999).

Cultural and religious beliefs and requirements, as well as personal values and experiences, influence someone's attitudes to their illness and to certain investigations and treatments. South Asian people who observe a strict code of modesty and are unwilling to undress or be touched, especially by a member of the opposite sex, can make the process of examination very difficult. It is important to understand the depth of distress and humiliation that exposure and physical contact can cause and to try and understand the patient/client 's point of view. Henley (1982) advises consideration of the following points:

- Expose only a small part of the body at a time, keeping all other parts covered.
- Ensure all windows and doors are closed or screened, and bed curtains are drawn.
- Wherever possible have a health professional of the same sex to carry out the investigations.
- Ensure that only essential people are present.

Ensuring respect for these concerns may require a little more time in planning and delivering care. The routine time frame of the coronary care unit (CCU) should not be allowed to unthinkingly override the needs of the patient.

Certain investigations and treatments may be difficult at certain times of the Muslim calendar. For example, during the Ramadan fast Muslim people may refuse to have blood taken in case they become weak. They may also be reluctant to take medications while fasting or to have investigations that involve eating and drinking (glucose tolerance tests and barium meals).

Confidentiality is very important to South Asian people too. It is essential never to assume that they have told their families about what is happening to them or details about their diagnosis, because they may not wish their immediate families to know. In a situation where someone declines to give consent for a procedure or treatment, especially when the illness is life threatening, it is important to find out their reasons sensitively and to see whether an alternative way forward can be found.

Health professionals have the difficult job of telling a person the truth about their diagnosis and prognosis. Whether people want to be told their diagnosis is influenced by cultural and religious beliefs (Henley, 1982). The Nursing and Midwifery Council (NMC) incorporates the shared values of respecting the person as an individual, obtaining consent for treatment, and protecting confidential information. Working within the guidelines of the NMC requires nurses to ensure that in times of conflict they are first and foremost accountable to the patient/client (Nursing and Midwifery, 2002).

Henley (1982) advocates the following principles in difficult and painful situations:

- Share a commitment to a duty of care, to patient autonomy, confidentially and consent, and to responding honestly to patients (for example, giving bad news).
- Understand the importance of respecting different cultural and religious values as part of the duty of care to patients.
- Keep well informed of the needs of patients and relatives, and their wishes and desires for knowledge of diagnoses, prognoses and available treatment options.
- Explain all reasons and actions to the relatives and patients.
- Give support to relatives whose wishes conflict with the professional's understanding of what the patient wants.

In seeking to fulfil these obligations it is appropriate to bear in mind how the patient understands the nature and cause of their illness, and what they regard as the appropriate treatment. The patient's health beliefs may powerfully impact upon how they respond to the diagnosis and how they conceive of their role in shaping their recovery. How individuals and communities perceive the nature of their illness, and how they understand their appropriate response to it has a major impact upon the process of care. An illustrative comparative example can be found in relation to the response to disability.

Background information on coronary heart disease

Coronary heart disease is one of the leading causes of death worldwide. It accounts for over six million deaths globally and in the UK is the commonest cause of death, accounting for over 125 000 deaths in 2000 alone (Petersen, Peto and Rayner, 2004). Although it affects both men and women, the figures suggest that one in four men will die from the disease as opposed to one in six women. An important feature of coronary heart disease in the UK is its unequal distribution in the population – death rates are significantly higher in manual workers than in professional groups. Ethnic differences have also been noted. People living in the UK whose ethnic origin is South Asian (from India, Bangladesh, Pakistan and Sri Lanka) have mortality rates 46% greater in men and 51% greater in women than the national average (Wild and McKeigue, 1997).

Coronary heart disease has a complex and multifactorial aetiology. Major risk factors include cigarette smoking, raised blood pressure, elevated levels of certain types of cholesterol, diabetes mellitus, and increasing age (Grundy *et al*, 1999). Genetic factors have also been shown to play a significant role in a person's risk of developing the disease, especially in the presence of other risk factors. Prevention involves paying attention to the risk factors, with regular monitoring for hypertension, cessation of smoking, preventing obesity, and monitoring blood cholesterol levels.

Hypertension, or high blood pressure, develops when the walls of the large arteries lose elasticity and become rigid, while the smaller arteries become constricted. Evidence suggests that people of African–Caribbean heritage are at higher risk of hypertension, as are people of South Asian heritage due to an increased risk of diabetes mellitus.

Monitoring of cholesterol levels is also important in prevention. Cholesterol is transported to the cells of the body via lipoproteins in the blood. Two main types of lipoprotein are responsible for transporting cholesterol around the body; these are low-density lipoproteins (LDL), or harmful lipoproteins, and high-density lipoproteins (HDL), or protective lipoproteins. The lower the density of the lipoprotein, the higher the fats contained within it. Triglycerides, which are found in fatty foods, are also responsible for increasing the risk of the disease. High tryglyceride levels are associated with obesity and high alcohol intake. Smoking is a well known to risk factor, whereby cigarettes contain chemicals such as carbon monoxide and nicotine that have a deleterious effect on the heart by increasing the viscosity of the blood, thus making the heart work harder. Other components of cigarettes, such as tar, are damaging in that they increase the build up of fatty substances within the arteries, adding to the risk of atherosclerosis. Excess weight has also been shown to increase the risk of the disease. It can cause the body to secrete hormones shown to be harmful to the circulatory system. Obesity also adds to the strain placed on joints and body organs, including the heart, and may lead to breathlessness, especially on exertion. Another well-known risk factor is diabetes mellitus, in which high blood glucose levels increase the risk of developing atherosclerosis. All the risk factors identified are compounded if there is a familial tendency or family history of coronary heart disease.

A major symptom of coronary heart disease is angina, which is caused by insufficient oxygen reaching the heart muscle due to a reduction in blood flow. Angina gives a sensation of heaviness, tightness or pain in the central chest area, which may extend to, or may just affect, the arms (especially the left arm), neck, jaw, face, back or abdomen. Angina is most often experienced during exertion, perhaps when running for a bus, playing a game such as tennis or football, climbing stairs, or walking uphill. An episode of angina may be precipitated by cold weather, ingestion of a heavy meal, or a stressful situations. The angina attack may subside once the precipitating activity ceases or on resting or taking medication. Some people suffering from the disease will experience a myocardial infarction or heart attack.

Infarction occurs when the blood supply to the heart muscle is interrupted or ceases, usually when a blood clot has formed or when the coronary artery is occluded or blocked or narrowed by deposits or atheromatous plaques (atherosclerosis). It causes severe pain, often experienced as a crushing sensation, or as a tight band around the chest. Unlike angina, this pain does not subside with cessation of activity or with rest. A number of other symptoms may accompany the chest pain, including sweating, light-headedness, nausea, vomiting, and breathlessness.

Transcultural nursing assessment of Mr Qureshi

In conjunction with the nursing process (assess, plan, implement, and evaluate) the acquisition of cultural knowledge ensures that culturally sensitive care underpins the plan of care that will be formulated for Mr Qureshi. The assessment that follows illustrates what information will be needed prior to developing an appropriate plan of care for him. The assessment of his needs is made by considering Roper's Twelve Activities of Living (Roper *et al*, 1983), by relating them to his normal routine. Any help or intervention from his caregivers (family members) is included where appropriate. Then the actual problems or reasons for intervention, along with recognition of any potential problems that may result from his physical or psychological needs, are examined.

Assessment of Mr Qureshi's care needs, showing the actual and potential problems he faces (within the framework of Roper's Activities of Living model)

Activities of living	Assessment of normal routine	Actual (A) problems and potential (P) problems
Maintaining a safe environment	Mr Qureshi lives in a close-knit Bangladeshi community, with his wife in a house that is shared with their eldest son and his family. He depends to a large extent on his family for his immediate care needs, including shopping for food, household items, and entertainment. He maintains an active role in the Bengali community, socialising with friend and neighbours	He will be unaccustomed to separation from his immediate family and members of the Bengali community of which he is familiar (A) He may be anxious about or frightened by unfamiliar figures (P) His family may be anxious about the impact of unfamiliar surroundings and language on his condition (P)
Communication	Mr Qureshi's first language is Bengali. He speaks very little English, relying on his son to communicate with people outside the Bengali community on his behalf. He takes regular medication for angina as and when required (self-administered). He is known to his family by a personal name (Khalid). He also has the religious name of Mohammed (not to be used alone)	He has a history of sudden-onset chest pain (A) He requires intensive cardiac monitoring, continuous observations of vital signs and further diagnostic tests (A) He may be unable to express his level of pain and may become agitated at his inability to communicate his needs to nursing staff in the absence of his family or an interpreter (P) He may be unused to or offended by inappropriate use of his name (P)

Activities of living	Assessment of normal routine	Actual (A) problems and potential (P) problems
Breathing	Mr Qureshi has experienced breathlessness on exertion	He is breathless and requires oxygen therapy (A) He may become agitated and anxious if oxygen therapy is increased or discontinued (P)
Eating and drinking	Mr Qureshi enjoys traditional Bengali cuisine, including meat, fish and vegetables such as cauliflower, aubergine and spinach. He enjoys drinking tea, and drinks no alcohol. His wife prepares his meals	He has an intravenous infusion in order to monitor fluid intake and administer medication (A) He only eats food prepared by his wife or immediate family (A) He may be unwilling/unable to eat food prepared by unfamiliar people (P) He may become malnourished while in hospital (P)
Eliminating	Mr Qureshi takes care of his elimination needs, requiring running water and facilities to wash his perineal area	He is confined to bed (A) He has a catheter inserted in order to monitor urine output (A) He may become agitated if he cannot attend to his elimination requirements, using running water (P) He may only accept assistance from immediate family members (P)
Personal cleansing and dressing	Mr Qureshi washes five times each day prior to praying. He maintains his own personal hygiene routine and requires running water	He is confined to bed (A) He may become agitated if he cannot access running water and wash prior to daily prayers (P) He will require assistance to wash and dress and may only accept this from immediate family members (P)

Activities of living	Assessment of normal routine	Actual (A) problems and potential (P) problems
Controlling body temperature	Mr Qureshi maintains his own body temperature. He has a tendency to feel cold due to lack of exercise as this often makes him breathless	He is confined to bed (A) He may feel cold due to lack of mobility, breathless on exertion, and oxygen therapy in situ (P)
Mobilising	Mr Qureshi does not usually mobilize well due to angina	He is confined to bed (A) Immobility may lead to increased risk of deep vein thrombosis, pulmonary embolism, and further myocardial infarction (P) He may not be able to communicate localised calf pain or increased chest pain (P)
Working and playing	Mr Qureshi is retired but takes an active part in the Bengali community of which he is a part.	He is unable to maintain links with friend and neighbours due to restricted visiting while in hospital (A) He may become isolated, lonely and anxious while away from his familiar community (P)
Expressing sexuality	Mr Qureshi is married, has one son and is a grandfather to three children	He will have restricted visitors in the acute stage of treatment for myocardial infarction (A) He may become isolated and anxious regarding his inability to maintain his usual position within the family (P)

Activities of living	Assessment of normal routine	Actual (A) problems and potential (P) problems
Sleeping	Mr Qureshi sleeps with his wife; he requires a firm mattress and four pillows	He suffers from breathlessness if in a prone position (A) He may be unable to maintain an upright poison in bed and may become breathless if in a prone position (P) He may have difficulty in communicating his need to remain upright in the absence of immediate family (P)
Dying	Mr Qureshi reads daily from the Qur'an. He has no fears about dying, as long as his family are with him. His family must be contacted immediately, if they are not present, and must be allowed to take care of his body, including washing, in the event of his death in hospital	He is acutely ill and in hospital (A) He may not recover or may suffer further myocardial infarction and may not survive (P) He may not have the opportunity to discuss his prognosis with nursing staff or family, in the event of a sudden deterioration in his condition (P)

Conclusions

In the previous chapter we looked at how research on ethnicity and health tends towards emphasis on genetic and cultural explanations (Nazroo, 1999). The reason for this is the way in which ethnic groups are identified in the research process, in spite of a general agreement that 'race' is a concept without scientific validity. The notion that people can be divided into races on the basis of genetic differences has been shown to be false (Barrot, 1996).

The case examined in this chapter takes account of, and is mindful of, the fact that there has been criticism of the well-publicised so-called greater risk for 'South Asians' in the UK of coronary heart disease as it relies on the misuse of 'race' as a way of identifying people for the purposes of research. The problem of coronary heart disease has been attributed to a combination of genetic (race) and cultural (ethnicity) factors that are apparently associated with being South Asian. Concerning genetics, there is a suggestion that South Asian people have a shared evolutionary history that involved adaptation to survival under conditions of periodic famine and low energy intake. This resulted in the development of insulin resistance syndrome, which apparently underlies the greater risk of the disease affecting them (Nazroo, 1999). Nazroo argues that by taking this perspective, South Asian people are being viewed as a genetically distinct group with a unique evolutionary history – a race. Furthermore, in terms of cultural factors, the use of ghee in cooking, a lack of physical exercise and a reluctance to use health services were all mentioned – even though ghee is not used by all the ethnic groups comprising the South Asian population, and evidence suggests that they do understand the importance of exercise and how to use the health services. The problem is apparently viewed as something inherent within a distinct biological group – it has nothing to do with the context of the lives of the South Asian population. Nazroo (1999) concludes that the tendency to view ethnicity in isolation leads to the racialisation of ethnic inequalities in health. Ahmad (1993) provides a robust critique of the simplistic use of consanguinity in the explanation of minority ethnic morbidity rates.

The assessment presented above draws on cultural knowledge of South Asian people, in particular those of the Muslim faith. A combination of culturally specific information with specific knowledge of coronary heart disease and myocardial infarction allows for a detailed assessment of actual and potential problems, which underpins a culturally sensitive and appropriate care plan.

CHAPTER 4

Children's Nursing

Children differ from adults, emotionally, physically, and intellectually. While it is clear that children have their own rights and deserve to have those rights respected in much the same way as adults, nevertheless children are vulnerable and can be at risk from dangerous situations and practices, as when suffering from ill-health, and/or when admitted to hospital. Children are protected by comprehensive legislation enshrined in Children Act 1989. This act provides the legal underpinning for the government paper *Every Child Matters: Change for Children* (Department for Education and Skills, 2004) – a programme aimed at transforming children's services. For more detailed information visit http://www.everychildmatters.gov.uk/. Children suffering from ill health and/or admitted to hospital are especially vulnerable if they belong to an ethnic group that is different to that of the care provider. This is because developmentally they, or their carers, may not be at a stage when they can 'make sense' of the world around them and the situation they find themselves in. This is compounded when their parents or significant carer is also compromised. This may be due to language/communication barriers, lack of knowledge of the health care system and processes, or lack of support from family members or friends. In many cases these problems will coexist. It is important to recognise that in making sure that treatment and care is the same for all children, and that discriminatory practice does not take place, we must also ensure that the individual needs of children from diverse ethnic and cultural backgrounds are recognised and respected, including the needs of the parents and/or carers.

This chapter aims to provide you with the skills required to nurse children from minority ethnic groups in a culturally competent manner. It will extend your understanding of how a nurse's knowledge of transcultural care can be transferred into practice in order to provide nursing care for children in a culturally sensitive manner. A number of cultural assessment models are available to assist in the implementation of the nursing process and can be adapted to fit the needs of the child (see *Chapter Three* for a detailed explanation). However, we need to be mindful of the particular needs of children in relation to a number of key concepts, namely independence/ dependence, communication, family relationships, health/ill health, and educational needs.

In order to apply theoretical principles to practice in relation to the transcultural care of the child, a case-study approach is used whereby a child of African–Caribbean heritage is admitted to hospital in crisis with sickle cell disorder. Knowledge of African–Caribbean culture is considered, and followed by a discussion of the condition of sickle cell disorder. A nursing assessment is then provided, which utilises knowledge of the child's cultural heritage and knowledge of the physiological illness. In this way, culturally sensitive care can be planned and implemented that recognises not only the child's health-care needs but also the cultural context in which the experience of ill health takes place.

Case study of Jasmine

Case introduction

Jasmine is a 6-year-old girl of African–Caribbean descent. She is admitted to hospital suffering from acute chest syndrome. This condition is similar to pneumonia, with symptoms such as difficulty breathing, chest pain and fever. Jasmine's acute chest syndrome has been caused by an infection and requires an emergency admission. In the A&E department Jasmine is assessed as requiring admission to the paediatric ward. She has received pain relief, antibiotics and oxygen therapy and is now in a stable condition. Jasmine now requires an assessment of her nursing and medical needs to manage her sickle cell disorder (SCD) while she is in hospital and in order to manage her ongoing healthcare needs on discharge from the acute-care setting. Jasmine has been accompanied into hospital by her mother who is very well-educated about the disease, as she is a sickle cell carrier, which means that she has inherited one gene for normal haemoglobin (A) and one gene for sickle haemoglobin (S). A person who has sickle cell trait (AS) is a carrier of the sickle gene, does not have the disease, and is generally not affected by the sickle haemoglobin. Sickle cell carriers are usually healthy (Sarjeant and Sarjeant, 2001). Jasmine's mother is used to caring for Jasmine including managing pain relief associated with SCD crises. Up to this point Jasmine has not needed to be hospitalised, consequently Jasmine's mother is concerned that the responsibility for care management will move from her to health-care professionals. She is concerned that the health-care staff will not fully understand the nature of pain associated with the disease. The nurse in hospital has the usual duties associated with caring for a child with a chronic disease that has acute, distressing episodes (France-Dawson, 1990), therefore it is important that health-care personnel have received training, which enables them to recognize and treat sickle cell crises and to reassure parent of children with sickle cell disorder that they have the relevant knowledge on which to base care. Jasmine's mother is also concerned that Jasmine will fall behind with her school work. It is a requirement of local hospitals to liaise with local education authorities to ensure that the educational attainment of a child with sickle cell is not compromised by hospital admission (Dick, 2007).

Background information on the cultural values, attitudes and beliefs of African–Caribbean people

The majority of people with 'Caribbean heritage' in the UK are primarily of African ancestry. However, because of the mixed ethnic population in the Caribbean, African–Caribbean people may be of Indian, Chinese and White British ancestry. Throughout the First and Second World Wars significant numbers of people came to the UK from the Caribbean. These older members of society will have been used to thinking of themselves as having 'island distinctions' and would have thought of themselves as Jamaicans, Begians or Trinidadians, for example.

In Great Britain, the term 'Caribbean' usually applies to the following islands, which were known as the British Colonies: Antigua, Barbados, Dominica, Grenada, Jamaica, Montserrat, St Kitts/Nevis/Anguilla, St Lucia, Trinidad and Tobago. However, it can also include the French islands of Guadeloupe and Martinique, Guyana on the mainland of South America, and other islands around the Caribbean Sea. The majority of African–Caribbean's have African roots, and in countries like Guyana and Trinidad, half the population is of Indian origin. In addition, there are White populations, mainly descendants of planters from colonising countries, and indentured labourers from Portugal and Spain, and people whose ancestors originated from China and Syria. These rich and diverse histories mean that African–Caribbean people have distinctive cuisines, stories, music and customs, which need to be recognised as playing an important part in the daily lives of individuals whether sick or well. Not to do so constitutes poor professional practice and leads to culturally inappropriate care.

The majority of African–Caribbean people born in the UK will have family and friends in Britain. Furthermore, their experiences will differ from those of their parents. However, the influence of culture on family does not diminish over time or place and this should be acknowledged when caring for children and families from other cultures, irrespective of place of birth. In addition, it is important to recognise that African–Caribbean or Black identity may take on different forms among British-born African–Caribbean people. It is important to note that a significant number of Black children in the UK have one White parent, including those of African–Caribbean heritage. Therefore, while an ethnic group may be defined as one that shares a common history, past or present, it should be noted that past and present has different meanings for different age groups.

As explained, African–Caribbean people are multiethnic–multicultural. This means that they may have different religions, languages, foods, art forms, music and social institutions or ideas, attitudes, beliefs, and values inherited from those who lived and are living in a particular Caribbean island. It is important to ascertain as much as possible from the child and family in order to plan culturally sensitive care. Ways in which cultural aspects of African–Caribbean life may diversify are discussed below.

Every island has its own distinct dishes associated with tradition and passed down through families. There is generally a strong influence from Africa, which forms the basis of Caribbean cuisine, for example the use cassava, cornmeal, sweet potato, yams, plantains, and okra in the daily diet. For some African–Caribbean people rice dishes may form the staple diet. Food may also be highly spiced and/or seasoned.

Religion may play an important part in the lives of some African–Caribbean people. A large proportion of African–Caribbean's are Christian, mostly of protestant denomination. Some are of Catholic faith and there are a growing number who follow Islam.

Caribbean languages have their origins in African languages, but the vocabulary used may be largely European in origin. African–Caribbean people have their own systems of meanings and rules of grammar. There is evidence of a level of debate within African–Caribbean communities around whether or not languages such as Jamaican or patois should be acknowledged as languages. However, it is important to acknowledge that for some people, a manner of speaking can be associated with social, educational, and financial success. In addition, a certain familiarity and use of African–Caribbean language can be an indicator of how 'in touch' a person is with their particular culture.

Associations between ethnicity and health status have been noted since quantitative health data were first recorded. However, it is often the case that conditions that are said to affect particular ethnic groups, such as African–Caribbean people, are not in themselves the cause of serious morbidity. While conditions such as sickle cell disorder can lead to serious ill health, there is a tendency to ignore differences in causes of ill health, which may affect certain ethnic groups more than others, economic factors being one such factor. The racialisation of research and health policy should be strongly resisted (Smith *et al*, 2000). However, many important determinants of health are physiological characteristics that are strongly influenced by socio-economic factors, and in turn have a long-lasting influence on health. Therefore, if a child with sickle cell disorder has to attend hospital appointments and suffers therefore from poor educational attainment because of 'lost' school days and the family cannot access help with this through lack of access to information and support, then the genetic predisposition of the African–Caribbean child to suffer from the disease is inextricably linked to the socio-economic and environmental situation of the child and family. The interrelationship between ethnicity, social position and health is complex, one which the health-care provider needs to be mindful of when making an assessment of the care needs of the child. Access to health care upon discharge may require assistance to be provided for travel costs. Health promotion advice, for example, extra nutritional supplements and a diet rich in minerals and vitamins needs to be given in light of the family or carers ability to finance this. Not addressing the financial position may lead to the family's growing sense of isolation and withdrawal from a recommended treatment programme, which may be construed as non-compliance.

Background information on sickle cell disorder

Sickle cell disorder is the collective name for a number of inherited blood conditions that mainly affect people of African, Caribbean, Middle Eastern, South Asian, Southeast Asian, and Mediterranean descent (Sarjeant and Sarjeant, 2001). It is also found in the Northern European population, albeit to a lesser extent (Dyson, 2005b). Sickle cell disorder affects haemoglobin, which is found in the erythrocytes (red blood cells). Two genes instruct the body how to make haemoglobin, one inherited from the mother and one from the father; normal haemoglobin is called haemoglobin A. An abnormal gene, however, instructs the body to make sickle haemoglobin, or haemoglobin S. If haemoglobin S genes are inherited from both parents, the child inherits sickle cell disease.

Haemoglobin serves to transport oxygen around the body. In this disease, however, haemoglobin S does not carry oxygen as well as it should, leading to the condition of anaemia, and with the result that those affected often feel tired and lethargic. For this reason, it is sometimes called sickle cell anaemia. Erythrocytes containing haemoglobin S don't work as well as ordinary erythrocytes because their normal shape (a 'ring doughnut') is affected. Under conditions of stress, which can be ill health, an inflammatory response, dehydration, a lack of oxygen as a result of excessive exercise or excessive cold, the cells can become distorted so they resemble a sickle or crescent shape (Meremikwu, 2006). Instead of being able to move freely through the blood vessels these 'sickled' cells can become lodged in small blood vessels so that blood is prevented from reaching some parts of the body, and causing moderate to excruciating pain. This condition is known as a sickle cell crisis. Children do not usually start to get attacks of sickle cell pain until they reach an age of three to six months, because fetal haemoglobin (haemoglobin F) protects babies both in utero and while they are very young. The effects of the disorder vary greatly from one child to another; some affected children are usually healthy, while others are frequently hospitalised. The case study described here is therefore not indicative of the experience of all children with the disorder.

To summarise, knowledge of the child's cultural background is a prerequisite to understanding the experience of ill health, in this case sickle cell disorder. In addition to the factors that impinge on the child's experience, for example, the frequency of sickle cell crises brought on by stress, infection, excessive exercise, and/or an overly cold environment, cultural factors also play a crucial part. The child with this disorder who learns to cope with the restrictions imposed by it, does so within the context of their cultural heritage, for example, the language used to express discomfort and pain, and the subsequent type of relief provided, often by parents and carers, that may be drawn from culturally derived practices. Often the strategies for relieving pain and discomfort are misconstrued by others (especially by teachers in school) as laziness or other so-called inappropriate behaviours.

Transcultural nursing assessment of Jasmine

Application of the nursing process (assess, plan, implement, and evaluate) and relevant cultural knowledge are needed to ensure Jasmine receives culturally sensitive care. They underpin the plan of care formulated for her. The detailed assessment below shows what information might be needed prior to developing an appropriate plan. The assessment is made within each of the twelve Activities of Living (Roper *et al*, 1983), and it includes details of Jasmine's normal routine, the help or intervention she gets from her mother, and the actual and potential problems she faces as a result of her physical or psychological needs, as well as reasons for any interventions.

Assessment of Jasmine's care needs, showing the actual and potential problems she faces (within the framework of Roper's Activities of Living model)

Activities of living	Assessment of normal routine	Actual (A) and potential (P) problems
Maintaining a safe environment	Jasmine depends on her mother primarily for maintenance of safety. Her mother has a detailed knowledge and understanding of sickle cell disorder, and usually administers all medication. Jasmine takes antibiotics regularly as prophylaxis	Jasmine will be unaccustomed to separation from parents or trusted adults (A) Jasmine may be anxious/frightened by unfamiliar figures (P) Jasmines mother is anxious about relinquishing care of Jasmine to nursing staff (A) Jasmine may not accept antibiotics or other prescribed medication from nursing staff (P)
Communication	Jasmine speaks English as a first language. Her language skills are commensurate with her age. Jasmine's mother often speaks patois. Jasmine often experiences pain associated with sickle cell disorder	Jasmine will be unfamiliar with terminology used to describe aspects of her care needs (A). She may be used to her condition referred to as sickle cell disorder, however the medical profession may refer to the condition as sickle cell disease. Jasmine and her mother may prefer the former to the latter Jasmine may be used to hearing some words spoken in patois (P) Jasmine is experiencing pain and requires pain relief (A) Jasmine may be reluctant or unable to express her pain level to unfamiliar nursing staff (P)
Breathing	Jasmine has sickle cell disorder. Her breathing is normally unaffected. However, she can become breathless on exertion and is prone to chest infection	Jasmine has acute chest syndrome on admission due to sickle cell disorder (A) Jasmine may develop respiratory failure (P)

Activities of living	Assessment of normal routine	Actual (A) and potential (P) problems
Eating and drinking	Jasmine has a normal diet with a preference for African–Caribbean dishes, including rice based dishes. Jasmine's mother is aware of dietary requirements in sickle cell disorder and liaises with the dietician regularly	Jasmine will be unprepared for food cooked in unfamiliar ways (A) Jasmine may be reluctant to eat unfamiliar food and may need extra calorific input (P)
Eliminating	Jasmine normally cares for herself, needing some help with access to toilet facilities and with removal of clothes. No nocturnal enuresis noted	Jasmine will be unfamiliar with her surroundings (A) Jasmine may be anxious/frightened and may not request help from nursing staff. Nocturnal enuresis may develop (P)
Personal cleansing and dressing	Jasmine can wash her face and hands. She needs help with bathing and dressing. This function is normally provided by her mother	Jasmine will require assistance to wash and dress (A). Jasmine may be anxious/frightened by being washed and dressed by nursing staff (P)
Controlling body temperature	Jasmine takes prophylactic antibiotics due to having sickle cell disorder	Jasmine is pyrexial on admission due to infection leading to acute chest syndrome (A) Antibiotic therapy may need review. Hydroxyurea may be prescribed (P)
Mobilising	Jasmine is normally fully mobile	Jasmine is immobile due to acute chest syndrome (A) Jasmine may develop enuresis, pressure sores, and may become irritable, anxious/frightened (P)

Activities of living	Assessment of normal routine	Actual (A) and potential (P) problems
Working and playing	Jasmine likes to play with friends and attends school	Jasmine is unable to socialise with her peer group and cannot attend mainstream school while in hospital (A) Inability to maintain normal developmental level (P) Isolation/regression/inability to engage in normal play activities (P)
Expressing sexuality	Jasmine likes to wear her own clothes and spend time with her mother	Jasmine will need to wear clothes with easy access for nursing/medical interventions (A) Jasmine may be anxious/frightened by unfamiliar clothing (P)
Sleeping	Jasmine normally sleeps through the night and sometimes requires rest in the day. Jasmine can become tired on exertion	Unfamiliar surroundings and stressful events may result in Jasmine becoming excessively tired (A) Jasmine is pyrexial on admission due to infection leading to acute chest syndrome (A) Jasmine may have disrupted sleep (P)
Dying	Jasmine does not normally express any concerns about dying. Jasmines mother is aware of the potential serious nature of sickle cell disorder and acute chest syndrome. Jasmine is Catholic but has not yet been confirmed	Acute chest syndrome is associated with mortality in children (A) Jasmine's mother may become anxious/frightened about the condition and Jasmine's prognosis (P) Jasmine's mother may require help and support from a Catholic priest (P)

Conclusions

Using the assessment in conjunction with guidelines for clinical care (see http://www.screening.nhs.uk/sickleandthal/ and info@sicklecellsociety.org) a plan of care can be produced for Jasmine, which takes into account not only her physical care needs but also her specific cultural care needs as a child of African–Caribbean heritage. The *Millennium Charter* (Action for Sick Children, 2000) summarises the important principles of child health based on the views of parents whose children are in receipt of health-care services (McEwan *et al*, 2003). Embedded within the charter is a requirement that all staff caring for children shall be specifically trained to understand and respond to their clinical, emotional, developmental, and cultural needs. By applying knowledge of the child's cultural heritage with a nursing model such as the Activities of Living model (Roper *et al*, 1983), the all important first stage in the nursing process (assessment) will take account of the cultural needs of the child and ensure culturally sensitive care is planned, implemented and evaluated.

CHAPTER 5

Mental Health Nursing

For the most part, people diagnosed with mental health conditions are cared for in the community. This situation is set to continue and indeed to increase given the demand on health-care resources and the growing trend generally to provide only the most acute care provision in a hospital setting. Where someone is admitted to hospital with a mental health condition it is likely that he or she will be discharged sooner than has been the case. The implications of this are that practitioners in the community need to ensure they have the skills to care for people from multicultural groups who may have mental health issues not previously encountered by the practitioner. An individual may have physical problems in addition to mental health conditions. Before considering best practice in assessing the health-care needs of people with mental health conditions from ethnic minority groups we need to understand something of the context of care for those who are suffering from mental ill health.

The distinction between illness and disease is an important one in that *illness* emphasises behavioural, psychological, socio-cultural, and experiential dimensions of disorders (Kavanagh, 2003). *Disease*, on the other hand, is the objective expression of a sickness, which manifests itself in chemical, physiologic, and other organic ways. A good deal of care given by nursing staff working in the field of mental health involves making daily life better and preventing illness for people with mental health disorders. Mental illness and mental disease are influenced by social and cultural factors. For example, a person suffering from loss of memory as a feature of a biological condition such as Alzheimer's disease will experience significantly less stress if cared for by a familiar person for as long as possible. Social arrangements for care may not alter the disease outcome for the sufferer. However, the illness trajectory may be positively influenced by familiar surroundings and faces. Similarly, cultural factors may positively influence the individual's experience of mental illness and disease. Diet, dress, language, and religious practice are all features of cultural life that are familiar and central to a person's sense of self, essence and well being. As such, cultural factors play an important role in the assessment of care needs for individuals with mental illness or disease in an acute-care setting and in the community.

All cultural groups share time-honoured systems of health beliefs and practices. Nurses working with different 'ethnic' groups should avoid a culture-bound approach that attempts to fit individuals into ready-made categories (Kavanagh, 2003). The use of models of nursing have been criticised for this reason, in that the temptation is to use the assessment framework of a given model in a rigid fashion, in the same way for each client. It is imperative to avoid a one-size-fits-all approach to assessment when a client has mental health issues. An individual may have an organic mental health condition similar to that of another person, but the individual's experience of that condition will vary greatly depending on socio-economic, environmental, physical and cultural factors. It is important, therefore, for the nurse to come to know who the client is, to understand the relationship that person shares with others, and to understand something of the nature of his or her world, including the environment in which they live and the influences on that life that make it unique. It is likely that the nurse and client will inhabit very different worlds, in respect of the cultural influences and the areas that impact on positive mental health, for example, migration history, educational status, and socio-economic status.

This chapter extends understanding of how a nurse's knowledge of transcultural care can be transferred into practice in order to provide nursing care for people with mental health conditions in a culturally sensitive manner. A number of cultural assessment models are available to assist in the implementation of the nursing process and can be adapted to fit the needs of this client group (see *Chapter Three* for detailed explanations). Issues of racism or stereotyping of ethnic groups as being more predisposed to certain mental health conditions are not considered here. For an excellent account of these important issues see Fernando (1995). There is no conclusive evidence that mental illness and disease rates vary between ethnic groups. What is clearer is the association of mental health issues with low socio-economic status, low educational level, separation, and loss. These factors are compounded for people, where English is not the first language, where carers communicate in English, and when interpretation services are not available or where the interpreter has little experience of working with people with mental health issues.

Transcultural nursing requires that nurses collect appropriate information about an individual's culture prior to undertaking the assessment stage of the nursing process. The cultural knowledge underpins the practice of undertaking the assessment. In addition to cultural knowledge the nurse needs also to understand the person's mental illness or disease in order to locate cultural factors within the context of his or hers condition. The case study below explains how culturally sensitive care can be provided for a man with Polish ancestry, who suffers with Alzheimer's disease

(Alzheimer's disease). It begins with an overview of Polish immigration to Great Britain followed by an account of Alzheimer's disease. In so doing, the care required can be located within a cultural, environmental and health-care context.

Case study of Mr Jerzy Wachowska

Case introduction

Jerzy Wachowska, a 77-year-old Polish gentleman, has been diagnosed with late-onset Alzheimer's disease, the symptoms of which include long- and short-term memory loss, feelings of agitation and anxiety, disrupted sleep patterns and an inability to make rational decisions. Mr Wachowska has recently suffered a fall, and has required outpatient treatment on four occasions for minor injuries from sharp objects, and on one occasion for a minor burn. He is increasingly incontinent of urine and faeces, which his wife claims are accidents due to poor mobility. If left unattended at meals times he sometimes chokes on large pieces of food. Mr Wachowska currently lives with his wife in a three-bedroomed house in a small Polish community, in a rural village. Village amenities include a supermarket, a GP surgery, a post office, a church, and a church hall, which also serves as a meeting place for members of the Polish club. The nearest hospital, with emergency facilities, is five miles away. He was a qualified teacher in Poland. He emigrated with his wife to the UK in 1950, for socio-economic reasons. However, in the UK he was unable to find employment as a teacher, working instead for thirty-five years, as a porter in the nearby hospital. He retired from this job, aged 60. Mr Wachowska and his wife have been, until recently, active members of the Polish club, meeting once a week to socialise with their community, who share many similar experiences of living and working in the UK in the post-war period. He has few friends outside this community and no living relatives in Poland. He and his wife have no family of their own; consequently, his wife has been his main carer since the onset of Alzheimer's disease. However, she now needs assistance from the primary health-care team so that she can continue to care for him at home.

Background information on the cultural values, attitudes and beliefs of Polish people

Since the date of Poland's accession to the European Union (1 May 2004) Polish people have been arriving in Great Britain in large numbers. Recent figures suggest they now comprise one of the largest ethnic groups in London with some districts now referred to as 'Polish towns'. London's conspicuously Polish characteristics now include not only people and language, but also a growing number of food stores, bookshops, restaurants, bars, and churches. In Britain as a whole, Polish immigrants belong to all social groups from business to student status. In spite of recent Polish immigration, which has seen an upsurge in the general debate about migration to Britain, it is important to remember that Polish people have a long history of migration to the UK and, indeed, to other parts of the world. Michalik and Konopnicka (2007) give a detailed account of the underlying reasons for, and trends in, Polish migration, some of which are summarised here.

Polish people constituted one of the largest groups of migrants from Eastern and Central Europe during the last century. Polish people have travelled to England and other parts of the UK throughout the centuries and their decisions to leave Poland were dictated by various needs and circumstances. Polish people migrated in search of labour and better living conditions, and to escape famine, disease and political persecution. In the sixteenth century Polish people came to England as traders and diplomats. In the eighteenth century the Counter-Reformation in Poland caused a small number of Polish Protestants to leave the country as religious refugees. The collapse of the November Uprising in the nineteenth century made many Polish fighters leave the country in search of refuge. However, the first large numbers of Polish people arrived in England, mostly settling in London, after the First World War.

The majority of Polish people came to England during the Second World War as political emigrants. In 1940, with the fall of France, the exiled Polish president, prime minister and government moved to London, with 20 000 soldiers and many other Polish people. London became the nerve centre and military headquarters of the Polish liberation movement. Towards the end of the Second World War, the resolutions of the Yalta conference led to the establishment of a Communist government in Poland, making many resident Polish people in Britain feel betrayed by their wartime allies. These Polish immigrants did not go back to Poland after 1945. Among this group, in addition to Polish military, were doctors, lawyers, judges and engineers, indeed very well qualified people. The relaxation of travel restrictions in Poland during the 1950s saw the number of people who decided to migrate to England steadily increasing. In 1991, in Poland, free elections of a Polish president led to the dissolution of the Polish government in London. For more than forty years the Polish people struggled hard to combat communism and gain one of the basic human rights – the right to liberty. Within a short time, London (which had been a base for the struggle against the communist regime in Poland) came to be seen as an important centre to develop political and business relations (Michalik and Konopnicka, 2007).

In the 1931 census there were 44 462 people living in Britain, claiming Poland as their birthplace. Those who arrived during the Second World War and stayed constitute the core of the present-day Polish community. In 1951 there were 162 339 Polish-born people in Britain. By 1971 the figure had dropped to 110 925. However, there are differences in the ways that Polish people have integrated and formed communities over time. There is evidence that more recent Polish immigrants are not as united as those who arrived in England after the Second World War. This could be due to the relative 'recentness' of their arrival in the UK, and the time needed for Polish communities to unite. Polish immigrants, like many other immigrant groups have to engage with finding employment and housing, leaving little time for social integration.

Today a significant number of Polish immigrants work in low-status sectors of the British economy. Some Polish immigrants have managed to find work in the professions for which they are qualified, for example, as doctors, teachers, or computer scientists. However, not all of those who have university qualifications find jobs in their fields as soon as they arrive in Britain, which could be due to few vacancies or language barriers.

When Poland joined the European Union in 2004, the people gained the right to work in some of the old EU member states. Great Britain (along with Sweden and Ireland) did not impose restrictions and, as a result, it has experienced a big and sudden influx of migrants from Poland. Statistics show that 264 560 migrant Polish workers, 82% of whom are aged 18–34, were registered in the UK by mid-2006. However, the number of actual immigrants is thought to be three times greater.

Although the immigrants were welcome at first, the fact that they arrived in such numbers and started to settle down all over the UK soon triggered a national debate. Some people argue that a Polish invasion of the British Isles is taking place, as not only London or bigger cities are the destinations of the immigrants, but also smaller towns and villages nationwide.

Generally, one can distinguish two opposing opinions concerning Polish workers in the UK. Clearly, they contribute to the economic growth of the country. They fill vacancies in the job market and are reliable and hard-working employees. Many Polish people take up the badly paid jobs that the British do not want (as happened with the Caribbean community who came to post-war Britain in the 1950s), as warehouse operatives, cleaners, domestic staff, care assistants and home carers, waiters and waitresses, bar staff, farm workers, kitchen and catering assistants, food processing operatives, construction workers, and drivers (see (http://www.uel.ac.uk/risingeast/currentissue/academic/). Moreover, despite well-recognised prejudice, Polish people are not a burden to state welfare. Michalek and Konopnicka (2007) write that by mid-2006, only 1.6% of national insurance numbers had been allocated to migrant workers from EU accession states. In fact, they even pay higher taxes: £112 per week as opposed to £100 paid by British nationals. Further arguments in favour of migration include the Bank of England statement that that the new wave of migration has been one factor preventing the rapid rise in oil prices from unleashing a damaging surge of inflation. Weaker inflation means interest rates can remain lower than otherwise (see http://www.workpermit.com/).

The opposing and clearly misguided view of UK citizens is that Polish people, and indeed other immigrants, are 'invaders' who steal jobs, drive wages down, and try to deprive rightful British citizens of their pensions and benefits. Further objections are that they bring their families with them and change not only the demographic structure of British society, but also its cultural traditions.

Background information on Alzheimer's disease

Alzheimer's disease is the most common form of dementia. It is a neurological disease, characterised by a loss of mental ability that can be severe enough to interfere with normal activities of living. For a positive diagnosis the condition needs to have persisted for more than six months and not to have been present from birth. The usual pattern is for it to occur in older age, with sufferers showing a marked decline in cognitive functions, such as remembering, reasoning and planning. A person with Alzheimer's will usually experience a gradual decline in mental functioning. This may begin with a loss of memory, which may be slight to moderate. Eventually the memory loss may impact on the individual's ability to maintain employment, to plan and carry out familiar tasks and activities, and to reason and exercise judgement. For some Alzheimer sufferers, mood swings and personality changes may be a feature of the condition. Evidence suggests that for most people diagnosed with Alzheimer's, death will occur within eight years of diagnosis (Cohen and Eisdorfer, 2001).

The causes are, at present, largely unknown. However, triggers are likely to be a combination of many interrelated factors, including genetic, environmental, and others that are not yet identified. What is clearer is that two types of Alzheimer's are seen: a rare autosomal dominant inherited *familial* form of the disease, and a *sporadic* form that has no obvious inheritance pattern (Geldmacher, 2001). It can also be described in terms of age at onset, with early onset occurring in people younger than sixty-five, and late onset occurring in those aged sixty-five and older. Evidence suggests that the early-onset form progresses more rapidly than the late-onset form.

Alzheimer's disease destroys neurons, or nerve cells, in the parts of the brain that are responsible for memory, such as the hippocampus, which is a structure that controls short-term memory. Once destroyed, the neurons stop functioning and short-term memory fails, along with the ability to perform familiar tasks. In the later stages of the disease, neurons in the cerebral cortex are affected, particularly the areas responsible for language and reasoning. When this occurs, language skills are lost and the ability to make judgements is affected (Mace and Rabbins, 2001). For some sufferers, personality changes are severe, possibly including emotional outbursts, wandering and agitation. As the disease progresses so does the severity of these distressing symptoms. Eventually many other parts of the brain become involved, brain regions atrophy (shrink) and the person may become bedridden, incontinent, helpless and non-responsive.

The symptoms begin gradually, most often with loss of memory. While occasional memory lapses are common to most 'healthy' people and do not signify any change in cognitive function, in the Alzheimer-affected person these memory lapses progress from the 'normal', perhaps just forgetting where the car keys have been placed, to the very severe, perhaps forgetting how to drive the car. The patient becomes disorientated, and may forget the names of family members and friends, or even forget the beginning of sentence by the time the end is heard. For an excellent account of the progression of the and the impact on the sufferers family, friends and carers read *Iris: A Memoir of Iris Murdock* written by her husband John Bayley.

As Alzheimer's progresses a number of other disturbing symptoms appear, including an inability to carry out routine and familiar tasks, and personality and behaviour changes. Some people may have trouble sleeping, and may become agitated in the evening. This distressing symptom is known as 'sunsetting' or 'sun-downer' syndrome. For some people with the disease, ideas, movements, words and thoughts are repeated. In the final stages of the disease, they may have severe problems with eating, communicating, and controlling bladder and bowel function (Sims, 2006).

Diagnosis is made through physical examination and taking of a medical history. History-taking needs also to include family members and caregivers as symptoms of Alzheimer's may be mimicked by using over-the-counter and prescription drugs. It is important to include in the assessment the usage of medicines, drugs, and alcohol, in order to exclude other causes of reported symptoms. Other medical conditions, such as tumours, infection, and other types of dementia (eg. mild stroke or mini-infarct dementia as a result of stroke) can give rise to Alzheimer-like symptoms. Blood tests, urine tests, brain magnetic resonance imaging (MRI), positron emission tomography (PET), or single photon emission computerised tomography (SPECT) tests may all be used to aid diagnosis. In addition, several oral and written tests are available to aid diagnosis and follow progression, including tests of mental status, functional abilities, memory and concentration. Early and accurate diagnosis is essential in developing management strategies and for ensuring that carers are given the support they need as soon as it becomes necessary.

At the current time, this disease is incurable. However, prompt intervention can slow decline from the disease and help sufferers to maintain independent function as long as possible. Medication can help (for an account of drug treatment for Alzheimer's see McReady, 2003). However, the remaining treatment is good nursing care, which provides for both the physical and emotional needs as they become more and more dependent and more erratic in their behaviour with progression of the disease. Modifications to the home may be necessary, possibly requiring assistance with financial and legal matters. Regular medical care is essential in order to avoid infections – a urinary tract infection may exacerbate the symptoms of Alzheimer's disease. It is important that any infection is diagnosed and treated correctly and not simply attributed to the inevitable decline associated with Alzheimer's (Mace and Rabbins, 2001).

In addition to the physical symptoms associated with this disease, sufferers may also become depressed and anxious and experience sleep deprivation. Each of these symptoms is, to some degree, treatable. However, it is perhaps most important to encourage the Alzheimer-sufferer to maintain a well-balanced diet and to take, as far as is possible, regular exercise. A calm, well-ordered environment is beneficial because it reduces anxiety and stress. In cases where psychiatric symptoms are manifest these may have to be treated with appropriate medication.

The person with Alzheimer's disease will gradually lose the ability to wash, dress, feed, bathe, use the toilet, and maintain their own safety. In the later stages the ability to move and speak will diminish. Nursing care is fundamental in relation to assistance with activities of living. What is more demanding and difficult is dealing with the unpredictability that Alzheimer's gives rise to in sufferers. At times this unpredictability due to erratic behaviour may lead to dangerous and at times inappropriate behaviour, which may or may not be of a sexual nature. Dealing with incontinence is a major part of nursing care, especially in the later stages of the disease, as is assisting with personal hygiene, feeding, and maintaining a safe environment, including prevention of falls, injection of poisonous substances, injury from sharp objects, fire or burns, and inability to respond to crisis situations. Giving medication and orientating the patient to time and place is another essential aspect of the nursing care.

Care for the caregivers is an essential part of the assessment of needs for the Alzheimer's sufferer. The care planned must take account of the fact that of all the dementias Alzheimer's places the largest burden on the carer. Carers will have experienced the impact of the disease on all aspects of their lives, from financial through to emotional. They may experience the whole range of emotions associated with caregiver-strain including mental and physical health problems, guilt, resentment, anxiety, sadness, and depression. Support for the carer is essential to enable their mental well being to be maintained, but also because of the positive impact on the patient from being close to and cared for by a familiar person.

To summarise, knowledge of the patient's cultural background is a prerequisite to understanding the person's experience of ill health, in this case Alzheimer's disease. In addition to the factors that impinge on his or her experience of the disease, already mentioned here – the importance of maintaining good physical health and the positive impact of familiar carers as apposed to unfamiliar care situations – cultural factors also play a crucial role in the trajectory of Alzheimer's. Diet, dress, religious practice and observance, and language factors, may in part, define an individual. The person with Alzheimer's who suffers memory loss, both short-term and long-term, may lose those aspects of their 'self' that have been central in maintaining a connection to their place of birth. This is especially true for immigrants to Great Britain. In this sense, the experience of 'taking away' away an individual's memories of time and place has a two-fold effect – not only does the disease decimate recent memories, but also memories of a life gone before.

The following nursing assessment shows how culturally sensitive care can be provided for Mr Wachowska, a man of Polish heritage who migrated to Britain in 1950 and who has been diagnosed with late-onset Alzheimer's disease.

Transcultural nursing assessment of Mr Wachowska

In conjunction with the nursing process (assess, plan, implement, and evaluate) the acquisition of cultural knowledge ensures that culturally sensitive care is behind the plan of care formulated for Mr Wachowska. The assessment below shows what information that may be needed prior to developing an appropriate plan of care for him. The first column details the twelve Activities of Living (Roper *et al*, 1983) within which the assessment of need is made. The second column details Mr Wachowska's normal routine within each activity, including details of any help and intervention from his caregiver, his wife. The third column details the actual problems he faces, or reasons for intervention, along with recognition of any potential problems that may result from his physical or psychological needs.

Assessment of Mr Wachowska's care needs, showing the actual and potential problems he faces (within the framework of Roper's Activities of Living model)

Activities of living	Assessment of normal routine	Actual (A) and potential (P) problems
Maintaining a safe environment	Mr Wachowska suffers from long-term and short-term memory loss due to Alzheimer's disease. He needs constant prompting and reminders to maintain health and safety inside and outside his home. His memory is better when he is in the company of his wife, as she is able to remind him of important key events and aspects of his life history	Mr Wachowska suffers acute memory loss (A) His memory will deteriorate in the absence of prompting and reminders from his wife (P) He is susceptible to falls and other injuries (P)
Communication	Mr Wachowska speaks very good English, but he often forgets conversations. He relies on his wife to remember details of conversations he's had with friends and neighbours from the Polish community	Mr Wachowska in increasingly unable to recall information (A) He may begin to communicate in his first language of Polish, as his short-term memory decreases and his ability for recall changes (P)
Breathing	Mr Wachowska is prone to chest infection due to difficulty mobilising and inappropriate dress. He often becomes agitated if made to wear clothing he does not like or is unfamiliar with	Mr Wachowska becomes agitated if made to wear unfamiliar clothing (A) He is at increased risk of chest infection (P)

Activities of living	Assessment of normal routine	Actual (A) and potential (P) problems
Eating and drinking	Mr Wachowska eats and drinks a normal diet, but needs assistance at times and requires all food to be presented in small amounts	Mr Wachowska will choke if left unattended at meal times (A) He may become agitated and aggressive if faced with unfamiliar carers at meal times (P)
Eliminating	Mr Wachowska is occasionally incontinent of urine and faeces if he cannot access the toilet in time	Mr Wachowska is doubly incontinent at times (A) Episodes of incontinence may increase as mobility decreases (P) Urinary tract infection, constipation, dehydration, agitation and aggression may develop as immobility increases (P)
Personal cleansing and dressing	Mr Wachowska needs assistance with washing and dressing. He often forgets where the bathroom and toilet are in his house. His ability to engage in washing and dressing is enhanced in familiar surroundings and with the assistance of his wife. His wife constantly talks about their life together in Poland as this helps to maintain a calm and secure atmosphere, while he is engaged in routine activities	Mr Wachowska cannot maintain an acceptable level of personal hygiene without assistance (A) His ability to engage in washing and dressing may deteriorate as his memory loss increases. He may become agitated at his inability to care for himself. He may be anxious if confronted by unfamiliar carers in his own home (P)

Activities of living	Assessment of normal routine	Actual (A) and potential (P) problems
Controlling body temperature	Mr Wachowska usually maintains his own body temperature, but recently he has been complaining of feeling cold. He regularly forgets to dress appropriately for the weather, and has been inclined to wander out of doors without suitable clothing	Mr Wachowska is at risk of reduced body temperature, due to inappropriate dress and inability to keep warm (A) He may become susceptible to falls or increases in environmental temperature, and be unable to adjust accordingly (P) He may become agitated due to increased body temperature or lethargic due to decreased body temperature (P)
Mobilising	Mr Wachowska mobilises with assistance from his wife. He is prone to falls due to unstable gait and unsteadiness	Mr Wachowska has difficulty mobilising (A) His mobility levels may decline, especially in the presence of unfamiliar carers (P) He may be at risk of deep vein thrombosis, and pulmonary embolism if immobility increases (P)
Working and playing	Mr Wachowska has been an active member of the Polish club. He is a qualified teacher, but has worked for thirty-five years as a porter in a local hospital. He usually socialises with friends from the Polish community	Mr Wachowska is unable to maintain his role within the Polish community (A) Lack of interaction with the Polish community mat precipitate further deterioration in his long- and short-term memory (P)

Activities of living	Assessment of normal routine	Actual (A) and potential (P) problems
Expressing sexuality	Mr Wachowska is married. He has no immediate family, apart from his wife, in the UK, and no remaining family in Poland. He enjoyed reminiscing with other male members of the Polish club	Mr Wachowska cannot attend the Polish club and often cannot remember other members names and faces (A) He may lose the capacity to remember his Polish cultural heritage, due to his inability to engage with his Polish compatriots (P)
Sleeping	Mr Wachowska has difficulty sleeping. He suffers from 'sundowners' syndrome, which leaves him anxious and agitated in the evening	Mr Wachowska exhibits agitation in the evening, which prevents him from sleeping (A) He may become aggressive, especially in the presence of unfamiliar carers (P) His sleep deprivation may become worse (P) He has an increased risk of falls due to over tired state (P)
Dying	Mr Wachowska has not expressed concerns about dying	Mr Wachowska has long-term and short-term memory loss (A) He may forget who his wife is (P) He may be unable to recall important conversations (P) He may forget important decisions regarding finances (P) He may forget important personal arrangements (P)

Conclusions

Mental health and mental illness are understood within the cultural contexts in which they develop (Gaines, 1992). Aspects of culture, such as diet, dress, religion, and language play a crucial role in determining how mental ill health is experienced. Often this information can only be gathered from family, friends and other carers. Holistic cultural care involves recognising the important contribution cultural heritage can play in mental well-being. The loss of long-term and short-term memory, such as occurs with Alzheimer's, compounds the sense of loss, not only for the patient, but also for family and friends, because it can signal the end of connections to a shared birth place and cultural heritage. For this reason, nurses engaged in caring for people with mental health needs, whether in the community or acute care setting; need to understand the cultural context in which they experience mental ill health. Nurses providing care to people with mental health conditions from different ethnic groups need to acquire knowledge of the special needs of the specific client group (Rajamanickam, 2007). Skills development is a prerequisite for culturally appropriate care and involves a knowledge of the client's cultural heritage as well as knowledge of his or her mental health illness. It is only when these dual aspects of essential knowledge are considered together that the nurse is delivering culturally competent care.

CHAPTER 6

Learning Disabilities Nursing

Learning disability is said to exist when people have a significantly reduced ability to understand new or complex information, learn new skills (impaired intelligence), or have a reduced ability to cope independently (impaired social functioning), which started before adulthood and has had a lasting effect on development (Department of Health, 2001). Precise figures on the number of people affected with a learning disability are difficult to ascertain. However, it is estimated that 210 000 people have learning disabilities, of whom 65 000 are children and young people, 120 000 are adults of working age, and 25 000 are older people.

The prevalence of severe and profound learning disability is evenly spread throughout the population and throughout different socio-economic groups. However, a mild to moderate learning disability is found to be more prevalent in deprived areas and has been linked with poverty rates. The number of people with severe learning disability in the population is set to increase by 1% over the next fifteen years for several reasons: increased life expectancy of people, especially those suffering from Down syndrome; growing numbers of children and young people surviving into adulthood with complex and multiple disabilities; the sharp rise in the reported number of school-age children with autistic spectrum disorders, some of whom will have learning disabilities; and the greater prevalence among some minority ethnic populations of South Asian origin (Department of Health, 2001).

There are many problems facing clients with learning disability and their carers. Many of these problems have their origins in social and political attitudes towards learning disability that include a lack of understanding of the range of disabilities and the individual needs of each person. Today the main problem is one of social exclusion. The Department of Health, in its comprehensive report *Valuing People: A New Strategy for Learning Disability for the 21st Century* (Department of Health, 2001) provides a detailed account of the issue of social exclusion for people with learning disabilities, covering such issues as the impact on families with disabled children, young disabled people at the point of transition to adult life, carers, choice and control, health care, housing, day services, social isolation, and employment. With respect to the needs of people with learning disabilities from minority ethnic groups, the report suggests this is an overlooked area, and makes the following key points:

- The prevalence of learning disabilities in some South Asian populations can be up to three times greater than in the general population.
- Diagnosis of learning disabilities is often made at a later age than in the general population and, as a whole, their parents receive less information about their child's condition and the support available.
- Social exclusion is made worse by language barriers and racism; negative stereotypes and attitudes contribute to the disadvantage.
- Carers who do not speak English receive less information about their support role and experience high levels of stress.
- Agencies often underestimate attachments to cultural traditions and religious beliefs.

Cultural beliefs regarding disability

Disability is viewed as a punishment in certain cultures. A child or adult with a learning disability may be viewed as being cursed by a supreme being, or as a result of having sinned, or having violated a taboo (Andrews and Boyle, 2003). In some cultural groups, the affected child or adult can be seen as tangible evidence of divine displeasure. In many communities long and protracted discussions may take place regarding the perceived wrongs committed by a family, and these are thought to manifest in the arrival of a disabled child. Such beliefs are covered in Anne Fadiman's (1997) book *The Spirit Catches You and You fall Down*).

Inherited disorders are considered by some cultures to be caused by a family curse that is passed down the generations through the blood-line. For families from cultures where this is the case, the nurse who attempts to establish carrier status for a particular inherited condition (sickle cell disorder and thalassaemia, for example) might be regarded as trying to determine who is 'at fault'. He or she may meet with resistance or anger when pursuing this line of enquiry by taking a genetic history. For more information, refer to Simon Dyson's book *Ethnicity and Screening for Sickle Cell/Thalassaemia: Lessons for Practice from the Voices of Experience* (Dyson, 2005).

In some Southeast Asian cultures a belief in reincarnation can lead to disability being viewed as evidence of transgression in a previous life, on the part of the parents of, or the child with, a disability. This may lead those parents to avoid seeking help or contact with support services for fear of recrimination and subsequent discrimination. In certain cultures disabled children and adults and their parents are avoided or discounted because of their perceived past lives and are encouraged to lead particularly virtuous lives 'this time around' to make up for their past transgressions. This can result in those families being ostracised from the community, with subsequent isolation and lack of care and appropriate support. In many cases the cultural attitude towards disability is so deeply embedded that even when genetic patterns of inheritance are explained to the family, the predominant belief is retained (Andrews and Boyle, 2003).

It is important that nurses who care for children or adults with a learning disability take account of the cultural heritage of the person affected and that of their carers. Ethnicity, cultural traditions, social and economic situations, living arrangements, employment status, and migration history are all contributory factors to the way in which disability and subsequent contact with health care and social services is experienced.

This chapter extends understanding of how a nurse's knowledge of transcultural care can be transferred into practice in order to provide nursing care for people with learning disabilities in a culturally sensitive manner. Several cultural assessment models are available to assist in the implementation of the nursing process and can be adapted to fit the needs of individuals with learning disabilities (see *Chapter Three* for a detailed explanation).

Transcultural nursing requires that nurses collect appropriate information about the individual's culture prior to the assessment stage of the nursing process. Such cultural knowledge underpins the practice of undertaking the assessment. As well as this cultural knowledge, the nurse needs to understand about the specific learning disability so that cultural factors can be located within the context of the client's condition. The case study explored below explains how culturally sensitive care can be provided for a family of Southeast Asian ancestry whose daughter has autism and associated learning disabilities. It begins with an overview of Southeast Asian culture and is followed by an account of the autistic condition, including its impact on the family. In this way, the care required by the learning disabled child can be located within a cultural, environmental and health-care context.

Case study of Mai

Case introduction

Mai Le, a 12-year-old girl, was born in the UK to Vietnamese parents. She has autism and associated learning disabilities. Mai is admitted to hospital suffering from severe abdominal pain and vomiting. A diagnosis of acute appendicitis is

contd./..

made and Mai is to be prepared for emergency surgery for appendicectomy. Mai is accompanied by her parents who describe their daughter's abdominal pain as commencing in the early hours of the morning. Mai's parents initially hoped the pain would subside and applied warm compresses to her abdomen. However, with the onset of nausea and vomiting they recognised the need to call for assistance, and one of their neighbour's called the emergency services. Mai is distressed and in considerable pain, which she expresses by rocking back and forth and crying. Mai and her family live in a small Vietnamese community within a large British city where they maintain the traditions of Vietnamese culture. Up to this point, the family have managed to care for Mai within their community, with minimal intervention from health and social-care services. Mai's parents speak a limited amount of English and do not appear to understand the complexity of the British health and social service systems, relying on neighbours to assist them in caring for Mai, which includes ensuring she is safe at all times. Mai attends a school for learning-disabled children where, in order to interact and socialise with other adults and children within the confines of her autism, she has to adhere to a particular routine each day. This includes regular meal times, familiar faces, restricted menus, and a regulated classroom environment. Any deviation from the normal routine is likely to cause Mai anxiety and result in disruptive and uncontrolled behaviour.

Background information on the cultural values, attitudes and beliefs of Vietnamese people

Vietnam, officially known as the Socialist Republic of Vietnam, is the most easterly nation on the peninsula of IndoChina. To the north, Vietnam borders China, with Laos to the northwest and Cambodia to the southwest. On the east coast is the South China Sea. Vietnam is recorded as having a population of over 85 million, which makes it the most densely populated nation in Southeast Asia. According to government figures for 2006, the gross domestic product (GDP) was 8.17%, giving Vietnam the second fastest growth rate among countries in East and Southeast Asia. For this reason, Vietnam is listed as being among the emerging economies.

At the 2001 UK census 22 954 Vietnamese-born people were recorded as living in England and Wales. The lack of a distinct Vietnamese category on the form (see *Appendix*) makes explicit information about the UK-born population difficult to ascertain. However, community organisations estimate that 55 000 live in England and Wales, of which 20 000 are undocumented migrants and 5000 are overseas students. Some 60% of Vietnamese-born people in England and Wales live in London (Sims, 2007).

The first refugees from Vietnam came to the UK between 1975 and 1981, most of them from North Vietnam (and ethnically Chinese). During the 1980s there was a second migration as families sought reunification. Most of these migrants were uneducated, had few transferable skills, and did not speak English – with obvious consequences for employment opportunities (Sims, 2007). Over the last five years, these immigrants have mastered the English language, so their employment opportunities have increased, especially in catering. However, there is still a high level of unemployment among these Vietnamese communities in some inner-city areas.

In the early years of migration Vietnamese resettlement studies showed that a high proportion of people were unable to speak English, a male bias in formal educational participation, and a population whose educational qualifications were generally low. On all these counts, there have been notable changes. The proportion of people admitting they cannot speak any English has dropped from 90% to 14%, although older people are disenchanted about the possibility of improvement, something indicated by the drop in language school attendance by this sector of the population. However, the overall picture of English language acquisition is of rapid progress, particularly among women. Females are now attending secondary and higher education in equal proportions to males negating the pre-existing male bias.

In relation to health status in Great Britain, evidence from the Policy Research on Ageing and Ethnicity (PRIAE) suggests that the elderly Vietnamese people suffer high incidences of osteoporosis and memory problems (PRIAE, 2005). The inability of early migrants to speak English resulted in a lack of knowledge of relevant social welfare allowances and had severe consequences on their ability access health and social-care services. This was coupled with a lack of knowledge and understanding of their culture on the part of health-care professionals, and contributed to this lack of support. Financial, housing, and educational difficulties compound the problems facing them in gaining access to health-care services.

Most Vietnamese people in the UK are ethnically Chinese. Nevertheless, there is a definite distinction between the Chinese and the Vietnamese communities in the UK, which are often seen as being diametrically opposed. Reasons for this may include the political context of the Vietnamese flight from Vietnam. Vietnamese migrants in the UK were seen as refugees and not, strictly speaking, immigrants, whereas the Chinese migrants were seen as immigrants from Hong Kong, or students. They are reported to have maintained strong business networks and close contact with the Chinese embassy, a resource that the so-called Vietnamese refugees were unable to call upon. In addition, the Chinese community in the UK has a long history, which the Vietnamese community does not.

In effect, Vietnamese in the UK are not monitored by the government as a settled minority (Sims, 2007). Only a few studies have taken place into the experience of the early immigrants to the UK. However, it is safe to say that they arrived as refugees under unfavourable economic conditions, with most being from rural backgrounds. The conditions they found themselves in would have been extremely socially challenging, involving a completely new language and culture. Once in the UK it is likely that they would have been forcibly dispersed around the country into what were effectively pockets of isolation.

The philosophy of life of Vietnamese people bears the deep imprint of the various religions in the country. The two main faiths of Vietnamese people are Buddhism and Christianity, although a number of cultural beliefs and practices are rooted in Confucianism, Buddhism, and Taoism. Confucianism sees the family as being first over all other commitments; as such, the westernised British view of individual freedom and choice can lead to cultural dilemmas for Vietnamese people, who may feel torn between adopting the 'British way' and maintaining their traditional cultural practices. The impact of this is more likely to be felt by second-generation Vietnamese – because they are born and educated within the British system they may experience conflict between the values and attitudes of their parents and the beliefs and practices of their British counterparts. Evidence suggests that many older Vietnamese people feel their traditional cultural heritage is becoming extinct (Sims, 2007). While Confucianism pervades the thinking of Vietnamese people from all walks of life, they do not follow all the tenets of the faith. For example, with regards to the lack of recognition for the authority of the female figure, when a father dies within a Vietnamese family, the mother does not have to obey the oldest male child; rather, the children continue to obey and respect her. The Buddhist influence can be discerned in the view of life on earth as something that is transient and unstable, whereby life may be viewed as an empty dream, in which all worldly riches, honours, and positions are temporary. Vietnamese people have an attitude of acceptance towards life that amounts almost to stoicism, with a general acceptance of their fate, whatever it might be. This attitude of self-contentment reflects the Taoist view of life.

In general, Vietnamese people tend to believe in the supreme power of the creator. This creator has no earthly origin or connection. No one can see the creator, although the creator sees everyone and knows everything. The creator is full of mercy and provides for each person his or her share of food and happiness. The creator rewards virtues and punishes sins. An individual may evade man-made laws, but may never evade the fair judgement of the creator. While Vietnamese people generally believe in the presence of fate in their lives, individual effort and enterprise can bring about change for the better. In relation to death, they believe that death is not total disappearance, however it is shrouded in mystery and, as such, life is always better. They believe there is a series of reincarnations after death, whereby the corporeal body dies but the spirits lives on. This belief in the survival of the soul leads to a feeling of gratitude and worship of their ancestors. The institution of ancestor worship, which bears witness to the influence of Confucianism on this culture, reflects their profound desire to survive in the heart and memory of loved one's after they have died.

Ancestor worship is shared by Vietnamese people of all faiths, except perhaps the converts to Christianity. Most families have an ancestral altar placed in a prominent place in the main room of the house. The ancestral altar is set with incense burners and candlesticks, together with the ancestral tablets and pictures. The head of the family is responsible for the proper veneration of the dead ancestors. On the anniversary of the death of each ancestor, special rites are performed. These rites consist of making offerings of sacrifice, burning incense, bowing and praying before the altar. This is an occasion for members of the family, relatives, and even close friends to gather together and have good food and wine. Besides the individual anniversaries of death, sacrifices are offered to the ancestors on holidays such as New Year's Day, the mid-Autumn Festival, and All Soul's Day. Whenever there is an occasion of family joy or sorrow, a wedding, a birth, a promotion or a funeral, rites are performed to honour the ancestors and inform them of the special event.

In relation to personal attitudes and beliefs, the Vietnamese culture places a high value on respect for self and others. Vietnamese are expected to show respect to those more senior than themselves and for those in a position of authority, within or without the family. Respect is shown through politeness, obedience and descriptive forms of address. In order to avoid embarrassment, Vietnamese people tend to avoid conflict, to hide their feelings and reject confrontation. The work 'Yes' may be used to signify the affirmative, but also as a device to avoid hurting the feelings of the other. They usually smile to avoid hurting the feelings of others when they do not wish to answer an embarrassing question, or when they have been admonished by an older person, in order to show that no offence has been taken. This type of cultural behaviour may be misinterpreted within British culture as representing a lack of engagement with officials in a given context, or even as insulting or challenging, depending on the situation. The phrase 'Thank you' is not overly used by Vietnamese people because it is deemed insincere. In the British cultural context, this apparent lack of gratitude may be perceived as rudeness. Another important feature of Vietnamese culture is the value placed on friendship. Visitors are always made welcome at any time of day or night. An expectation that this easy and open attitude towards visiting will be reciprocated may have implications for compliance with hospital visiting times, arising through a lack of understanding of the reasons for restricted access to their loved ones. Self-respect and 'saving face' are important cultural features too. Self-respect, once lost, is hard to regain for Vietnamese people. Hurt feelings tend to remain in the memory for considerable time and lost confidence, whether in an individual or an organisation, is hard to regain.

Another significant cultural factor is the attitude towards time-keeping. Punctuality may be good, but some Vietnamese tend to have a more relaxed approach to time keeping, often involving a ten-minute leeway, which may have implications for hospital appointments or outpatient appointments at clinics.

As regards the physical aspects of care that may be required in the course of treatment, Vietnamese people do not like to be touched by members of the opposite sex. Certain touching practices like touching the head, are not allowed except in the case of small children. Gesturing or calling someone using an index finger is considered rude.

The Vietnamese diet is richly influenced by the cuisine of France, China, and Thailand. Vietnamese cuisine consists of the use of herbs such as lemon grass, coriander, and parsley, and key ingredients are laksa leaf, lime and chilli. Most meals include soup. Snacks often include spring rolls and rice cakes. A piquant spicy fish sauce called *nuoc mam* is a served with most meals.

Background information on autism

Autism is a developmental disorder that results in a cluster of abnormal behaviours. It affects children from birth or their early months and leads to deviations from normal behaviour patterns in three areas:

- Social relations and interactions
- Language and communication
- Activities and interests.

When the triad of developmental problems occur, beyond the patterns of deviation seen in normal childhood behaviour, autism is said to exist.

An agreement about the terms and definitions for autism has led to children who exhibit problems in these three areas of development being diagnosed with autism spectrum disorder. Further tests are available that can specify additional features of the condition, such as its severity, the cognitive level, clinical traits and associated medical conditions (Gillberg, 1990). Although autism itself is more than likely present from birth, or very soon afterwards, the nature of the condition means that some developmental features do not become apparent for months or even years.

The incidence of autism is difficult to establish due to problems of diagnosis. However, the National Autistic Society (1997) estimates a prevalence rate of 1 in 100 people in the UK with autistic spectrum disorder.

The cause of autism is as yet unknown, although most clinicians believe the condition originates from some sort of brain injury, possibly prenatally. Contributing factors may include genetic or chromosome abnormalities, viral agents, metabolic disorders, immune intolerance, and perinatal anoxia (Humphries, 2007). These factors explain why children diagnosed with autism can have additional learning disabilities. However, this is not a full explanation – there are brain injured children who do not go on to develop autism.

In some cases there is no apparent cause for childhood autism. However, what seems clear, irrespective of the origin of the autism, is a final common pathway that results in difficulties in social communication and obsessional traits, and/or learning disabilities (slower development in almost all areas), with a degree of overlap in some cases (Baron-Cohen and Bolton, 1993).

Diagnosis of autism before the age of two is unusual. In most cases it comes much later. Comprehensive, specialist assessment is essential and requires the primary health-care team (GPs, community health specialist practitioners) to be aware of and alert to the features of autism in children. Early recognition allows families to access the support they need and helps them to respond and adjust to their child's special needs. In the case where the child has learning disabilities in addition to autism, the community nurses working with learning-disabled people may be the first to suspect autism is present. Health visitors and community paediatric nurses may also be involved in the management of autistic children.

Parents of children with autism may, in the first instance, recognise their child as being 'different' from other children of a similar age. However, quite often parents are unable to articulate what this difference actually is. This requires all health-care professionals to pay attention to the concerns expressed by parents, irrespective of how imprecise they might at first appear (Humphries, 2007). For some parents of children with autism, nothing untoward is noticed. This may be due to poor knowledge of childhood developmental milestones or few opportunities for comparison, or because they have little access to child development texts and information, or a because they are disinclined to recognise or distinguish behaviour as deviating from the 'normal'.

Recognition of autistic characteristics is difficult in the early months of childhood, hence the reasons for later diagnosis. However, there are characteristics that suggest autism is present. Wing (1980) identified two types of autism in the child: the placid, undemanding baby who rarely cries, and the reverse, or screaming, baby who is difficult to pacify. Babies, she notes, may rock, or bang their heads, or scratch or tap at their blankets when in their pram or cot, or develop a fascination for shiny twinkling objects. They may have an apparent lack of interest in people, animals or traffic. These behaviours may be displayed by children who are not affected by autism, or by children with some learning disability other than autism. Therefore caution is needed before interpreting such behaviours as indicative of autism.

Symptoms of autism are varied and may include peculiarities of hearing, so that the child is suspected of being deaf from an early age. Very rarely is a child with autism deaf, even though they may well not respond to their name and appear unaffected by audible changes in their environment. Autistic children may appear to ignore the loudest of noises, ones that would be expected to startle other children. In addition, children with autism may be drawn to certain sounds from a considerable distance, such as those made by a friction-driven toy or a sweet being unwrapped. Other sounds may cause extreme distress, such as a police siren or a barking dog (Humphries, 2007).

Young babies affected by autism may show a lack of interest in the usual types of play enjoyed by infants at the same developmental stage, including those involving social interaction with their parents. This feature of autism can be extremely upsetting and disturbing for the parents, especially when they have other children for comparison, within and without the family. A lack of shared interest, an inability to actively partake in baby games, and an inability or disinclination to point out things of interest, are all reported features of autism in babies (Frith and Soares, 1993).

Early referral and assessment are key to the management of childhood autism and are best carried out at an appropriate childhood assessment centre. A variety of health-care professionals may need to be involved, using a team approach to diagnosis. Assessment demands an accurate family history, including antenatal history, the child's behavioural history and developmental progress. A physical assessment of the child is also important to determine the presence of underlying medical conditions that may contribute to deviations or developmental delay. Developmental assessment of the child will include fine and gross motor skills, language (reception, expression and verbalisation), sensory perception, social and emotional development, and play. The way skills are used by the child is as important as the presence of the skills. For example, a child with autism may have acquired the skills to reproduce words, but not have developed an understanding of their meaning (Baron-Cohen *et al*, 1992). The novel by Mark Haddon *The Curious Incident of the Dog in the Night Time* gives a thorough insight into this condition (Haddon, 2004).

There is no known cure for autism. Children with autism become adults with autism. Those with autism in addition to learning disabilities will require care and supervision for their whole lives. All interventions are designed to assist the affected person as a child and an adult, to achieve their full potential at all stages of their lives and to support and help their parents and carers to accomplish this (Humphries, 2007).

To summarise, knowledge of an individual's cultural heritage is an essential prerequisite for understanding the experience of hospitalisation, in this case for a child with autism who has associated learning disabilities. In addition to the factors that impinge on the experience of autism (early recognition, assessment and appropriate referral) cultural factors play a crucial part. Religious practice and observance, language factors, attitudes towards health-care providers and conventional forms of medicine will impact on the experience of emergency hospital admission. The ability to understand and engage with complex unfamiliar medical systems and health care-agencies compounds the difficulties and increases the likelihood of a traumatic experience. Being aware of and paying attention to the cultural factors that affect the individual's experience of health-care treatment is essential for the provision of culturally sensitive and appropriate care.

The nursing assessment that follows shows how culturally sensitive care can be provided for Mai, a young person of Vietnamese heritage who has autism and associated learning disabilities and is admitted to hospital as an emergency.

Transcultural nursing assessment of Mai

In conjunction with the nursing process (assess, plan, implement, and evaluate) acquisition of cultural knowledge ensures that culturally sensitive care underpins the plan of care formulated for Mai. The assessment below provides an example of the information needed prior to developing an appropriate plan of care. The twelve Activities of Living (Roper *et al*, 1983) within which the assessment of need is made are considered in turn, and considered in the context of Mai's normal routine, as well as the help and interventions received from her parents, as her caregivers. The actual problems and potential problem that could from Mai's physical or psychological needs are identified.

Assessment of Mai's care needs, showing the actual and potential problems she faces (within the framework of Roper's Activities of Living model)

Activities of living	Assessment of normal routine	Actual (A) and potential (P) problems
Maintaining a safe environment	Mai does not recognise dangerous situations. She has no understanding of potentially harmful appliances and no understanding of electricity, or extreme heat or cold	Mai is confined to bed rest (A) She will not understand the equipment surrounding the bed, or being used as part of treatment (oxygen, suction apparatus, intravenous infusion) (P)
Communication	Mai speaks English. She has a vocabulary consistent with her age. However, she does not always fully understand the meaning of words used. She is polite and respects all elders. She is unused to being overly touched and is not used to overt displays of affection	Mai is to be prepared for surgery for appendicectomy (A) She will not fully understand the meaning of informed consent (P) Her parents may not fully understand the meaning of informed consent (P)
Breathing	Mai can become breathless if agitated or upset. She has been known to hyperventilate in unfamiliar situations	Mai is in an extremely unfamiliar situation (A) She will be undergoing surgery for appendicectomy (A) She may become agitated and start to hyperventilate in unfamiliar situations (P) Her parents should be encouraged to accompany her to the operating theatre (P)

Activities of living	Assessment of normal routine	Actual (A) and potential (P) problems
Eating and drinking	Mai eats and drinks from a special plate, bowl and cup, using her own knife, fork and spoon, and becomes extremely agitated if these are not available. She does not like the colour orange and will therefore not eat orange food including carrots, orange jelly, oranges, orange marmalade, or drink orange juice. She eats food prepared by her parents, which is traditionally Vietnamese cuisine	Mai is 'nil by mouth' on admission, prior to surgery (A) She has an intravenous infusion in situ to alleviate and prevent dehydration (A) Her parents may not fully understand the treatment given (P) She may become agitated and try to remove the intravenous line (P)
Eliminating	Mai is continent, but in unfamiliar situations she has been known to become distressed and refuse to use toilet facilities that are unfamiliar to her. She has suffered from constipation on four occasions, which is usually relieved by an immediate return to normal routine and the resumption of normal dietary intake. She will not drink orange juice or eat oranges, but she will eat other fruit. She does not like taking medication	Mai is confined to bed rest prior to surgery (A) She will need to use a bed pan (A) She may not be used to unfamiliar equipment and/ or unfamiliar surroundings (P) She may become constipated and refuse medication for same (P) Her parents may not fully understand the requirement for bed-rest (P)

Activities of living	Assessment of normal routine	Actual (A) and potential (P) problems
Personal cleansing and dressing	Mai maintains a hygiene routine involving personal soap, toothbrush, and towels. She will not wash if unfamiliar articles are used and will not wear orange-coloured clothes. She likes to choose her own clothes each day	Mai is confined to bed-rest and is to be prepared for surgery (A)
Controlling body temperature	Mai does not recognise the implications of changes in temperature. She will not wear unfamiliar clothes. She prefers clothes made by her mother and likes traditional Vietnamese dress	Mai is to be prepared for surgery (A) She may have difficulty complying with preparations for surgery (P)
Mobilising	Mai does not like to be confined. She walks to school each day	Mai is confined to bed-rest (A) She may become irritable and attempt to mobilize (P)
Working and playing	Mai will only engage in certain types of play. She enjoys the company of some children and not others. Certain colours (orange) and certain noises can cause distress (whistles, loud bangs). Her school-teachers try to provide a routine each day. She enjoys the company of Vietnamese children in her school and community as they are familiar to her	Mai is confined to bed-rest prior to, and immediately after surgery (A) She may become withdrawn and anxious due to separation from friends and family (P)

Activities of living	Assessment of normal routine	Actual (A) and potential (P) problems
Expressing sexuality	Mai likes to dress in familiar clothes especially those made by her mother, which tend to be Vietnamese in style and texture. She does not like to be touched by adults she does not know because touching by people not familiar to the family is culturally inappropriate (may include health professionals if the family are unaware of their position and role in providing treatment and care)	Mai will be prepared for surgery (theatre clothing) (A) She may become anxious and uncooperative with preparation for surgery (P) She may be made anxious by physical assessment and examination if her family are not present (P) Her family may not fully understand the need for assessments and examinations (P)
Sleeping	Mai likes to sleep in her own bedroom with familiar items around her. She likes traditional Vietnamese toys, which she has had for a number of years	Mai will be in unfamiliar surrounding (A) She will be separated from her favourite toys for a short period of time (P) She may not sleep properly because of the unfamiliar people and surroundings (P)
Dying	Mai's family have strong views about death and dying which are culturally determined. Mai will have the same cultural heritage, but may not fully understand the concept of death	Mai has acute appendicitis (A) She may not fully understand the implications of non-compliance with treatment and medication (P)

Conclusions

This assessment highlights the complexities surrounding culturally sensitive care for people with learning disabilities, and their carers, not least those related to communication. The assessment of health-care needs must consider the client's and carers' cultural heritage(s) as an integral part. When this occurs it becomes clear that the wishes of the client, family and/or other carers are central to effective communication and successful treatment outcomes. However, on occasions the concerns and desires of the client and carers become secondary to the need for health-care professionals to carry out care, especially in the event of an emergency. In order to optimise recovery it is vital to recognise the role culture plays in recovery. Information concerning all aspects of care and treatment must be given in a meaningful way, in order that client and carers may fully understand the need for treatment and the implications of non-compliance with treatment. In this way the client and carer's can be enabled to make informed decisions about treatment. One way of maximising the effectiveness of communication is through the use of interpreters (see *Chapter Three*). However, it is often the case that access to interpretation is limited due to lack of resources. Furthermore, when interpretation services are available, the quality is often poor (Bradby, 2001). A different approach to ensuring that clients and their carers receive optimal care, including information, is to appoint a key worker to the family. However, recent research into the experiences of families where key workers have been appointed indicates that it should not be taken for granted that this measure solves all problems (Mir, 2007).

Health-care professionals can feel ill-equipped to respond to the needs of different ethnic groups and come to rely on co-workers who are of the same cultural heritage as the patient or client. While this may in some circumstances be appropriate, although never ideal because it can put strain on relationships that professionals have with each other and with their clients, it is made more difficult when the ethnicity of the client is one not encountered previously. Reliance on co-workers to interpret can lead to the assumption that the ethnicity of the client is the same as that of the professional, for reasons that the client and professional may share some similarities, perhaps in language, dress, and religion. The inability to recognise diversity within ethnic groups often causes deep distress to clients and professionals alike, and impacts on the way that clients experience health-care services in the future. Recognition of diversity within ethnic groups is key to providing culturally appropriate and sensitive care.

CHAPTER 7

Transcultural Nursing in the Nursing Curriculum

So far, in this book, we have considered the history of multicultural Great Britain as a means to understanding the diverse society we live in today. The importance of understanding our own cultural heritage as a prerequisite for understanding the cultural heritage of others has been emphasised as fundamental to the provision of culturally competent care. We have considered the importance of understanding the language and terminology used in learning, teaching, and practising the art of transcultural nursing through an examination of the concepts of 'race', ethnicity, ethnic minority, racism, human rights, and culture. If nurses are to provide sensitive and appropriate care for people from diverse ethnic groups it is essential to underpin practice with correct use of language. Not to do so can cause offence and lead to patient/clients and their carers losing faith and lacking trust in health-care services, which then has a detrimental effect on their recovery.

A number of transcultural nursing models have been reviewed (see *Chapter Two*). In doing so, no particular model is advocated, as the choice of model should be patient/client- and context-specific. Models of transcultural nursing can guide practice by drawing attention to the kinds of questions we should be asking that take account of cultural heritage and the role culture plays in individual experiences of ill health, both physical and psychological. When combined with detailed knowledge of the patient/client's disorder or disease an assessment of need is facilitated, which provides the basis for planning, delivering and evaluating culturally appropriate and competent care (see Chapters *Three, Four, Five,* and *Six*).

In an early section of this book we discussed emerging trends in transcultural nursing that have sought to enhance harmony in culturally diverse Great Britain. These include assimilation, whereby minority ethnic communities are encouraged to adopt the values of the society in which they find themselves; multiculturalism, whereby the promotion of understanding of cultural diversity underpins better understanding between cultural groups; anti-racism, which considers the polices and structures in society that may mitigate against cultural harmony; and a combined multicultural and anti-racist approach that moves us some way towards understanding that no single approach adequately explains the factors that precipitate racial disharmony and tension. The decision to focus on a particular approach to enhancing cultural harmony was made within the cultural knowledge available at the time. With hindsight, we are able to evaluate and recognise when approaches to transcultural care have been less than successful in meeting the needs of individuals from diverse ethnic groups.

This chapter looks at ways nurse educators can influence future directions for transcultural nursing through education.

Research and professional practice

One way to ensure practitioners are enabled to meet the needs of people in a multicultural society is by engaging nurses with research around ethnicity and health. This specialist field of research continues to develop and provides the way forward for more appropriate ways of caring for an ever increasing diverse population. Nursing research around ethnicity and ethnic health should be conducted in a culturally sensitive manner and should not be undertaken for its own sake, but rather to inform transcultural nursing practice. Culturally appropriate research can be problematic in that respondents may be poorly informed of the aims of the research, be unable to give informed consent, and feel unable to refuse to participate. Nurses need to be aware of the complexities around research with different ethnic groups and ensure that they have access to proper training in issues relating to culture and ethnicity (Papadopoulos and Lees, 2002). Proper research training enables nurses to avoid taking a unicultural perspective that assumes that concepts are universally applicable across cultures, as this curtails researchers' awareness of alternate interpretations. The issue of racialisation of ethnic inequalities in health is discussed by Nazroo (1999).

The complexities of research around ethnicity and ethnic health should not prevent nurses from engaging in culturally sensitive research. Evidence-based practice is as important in transcultural nursing as in other aspects of the art and science of nursing, such as clinical practice, the sociology and psychology of health and illness, anatomy and physiology, and ethical issues in health care. Practice is a central element of nursing, therefore practice-based research should underpin transcultural nursing practice. Too often nurses rely on research carried out in academic departments to underpin practice. While the quality of the research may be excellent, the practical application of the research should be the concern of practitioners.

Holland and Hogg (2001) provide a detailed account of cultural diversity and professional practice in which they look at the issues around the history of Black and minority ethnic nurses in the National Health Service. They indicate that racism in nursing practice is not new. This theme is also discussed by Culley and Dyson (2001). Most nurses will be aware of the Black nurse Mary Seacole, a contemporary of Florence Nightingale, whose work for the British Army during the Crimean War led to her recognition by Queen Victoria. What is not so well known is that Mary Seacole's account of racist practice detailed in her descriptions of how she was treated by others. Seacole clearly identified a change in attitude and behaviour towards her, which she attributed to a distaste and dislike of her skin colour on the part of the other nurses. Nurses should not be lulled into believing that accounts such as these are consigned to history and have no relevance for today's professional practice. On the contrary, recent research with Zimbabwean nurses living, working and studying in the UK found that racism continues to be a feature of the NHS (Dyson, 2005). The research respondents identified the perpetrators of racist practice as being practitioners, other students, and lecturers. Sadly, it is often the case that the perpetrators of racism do not understand the true meaning of racist practice and tend to minimise its impact. We have seen the recent debacle in the media caused by apparent racist behaviour on the part of a celebrity who appeared not to understand the implications of a particular form of language. It could be argued that lack of education is partly to blame for some forms of racist practice, in particular the use of inappropriate language. While this does not minimise the impact of racist practice it does go some way to explain why it can occur in some situations. Moreover, by recognising the implications of lack of education around what is and is not racist practice we are able to move towards a more coherent approach to promoting cultural harmony, and one which recognises the central role of education in changing behaviour. Culturally sensitive and appropriate nursing care can only be provided if nurses are competent to do so. Nurse educators responsible for undergraduate and postgraduate programmes must strive for quality within transcultural nursing education, by ensuring appropriate research, including research methods training around ethnicity and ethnic health are integral to the curriculum.

The use of transcultural nursing models in nurse education

Many models are available to assist in the process of incorporating transcultural nursing into the curriculum in a meaningful way. Consistent with the approach taken in this book, no ingle model is advocated. Instead, nurse educators are advised to choose the model that best facilitates the inclusion of transcultural education into their particular nursing programme, as this recognises that nursing programmes differ in educational philosophy, programme structure, process of delivery, and attainment level. Paula McGee (1992), drawing on the work of Byerly (1977), describes four broad approaches to incorporating transcultural education into the nursing curriculum. When considering the relevance of each approach, the philosophy underpinning the nursing programme needs to be considered in order to ensure the best 'fit'. Each approach is described with additional commentary on how they may be incorporated in to different types of nursing programme.

The integrative approach

In the integrative approach transcultural concepts pervade the whole curriculum: cultural concepts and constructs are unified with other content; students discover, create and think about cultural issues rather than gather facts. An integrated approach may be best where a spiral curriculum guides programme delivery. The spiral curriculum, originally developed by Bruner in 1960 sees students coming round through a series of themes and returning to familiar concepts and ideas presented at increasing levels of difficulty and which the curriculum presents using a variety of samples (Bruner, 1960). In this approach students revisit familiar theory and practice, but each successive experience builds up and each topic is gone into more broadly and at a greater depth and difficulty (Greaves, 1987). Where a spiral curriculum underpins the nursing programme, an integrated approach to transcultural education would allow for cultural concepts and constructs to be taught alongside other subjects and returned to at appropriate points. As students progress through the programme transcultural education is returned to in the context of the students' clinical practice and taught theory. In this way the cultural education is meaningful and relevant to the students' experience.

The unit-construction approach

In this approach, specific learning units deal primarily with cultural concepts in health and nursing care. Each component of the nursing curriculum, whether child health or care of people with learning disabilities includes a unit of study on related transcultural concepts. A unit-construction approach may be best suited where a core-curriculum approach is taken to programme delivery. Core curriculum concentrates on functions, problems, or situations (Taba, 1962; Wheeler, 1967). The aim of a core-curriculum approach is to promote unity of content and meet the needs common to all students on the nursing programme. There is generally an attempt, when using a core curriculum approach, to break down the traditional subject division boundaries that exist between disciplines and in order to do this the core programme combines with other courses or elective options (Greaves, 1987). Where core curriculum underpins programme delivery a unit-construction approach to transcultural education would allow specific units of cultural education to be included in each core component of the programme. For example, a core research component would include research around ethnicity and ethnic health.

The course approach

A course approach is one in which 'educationally prepared' teaching staff are responsible for the delivery of transcultural education (with a background in anthropology) within the nursing programme to provide concentrated emphasis on cultural aspects of health and illness. Where nursing programmes draw on teaching staff across disciplines within and outside nursing (sociologists, psychologists, medical practitioners, biologists, etc.) the course approach may be appropriate. Cultural aspects of health and illness would be taught by academics in the field of ethnicity and ethnic health in the same way that other aspects of the programme are taught by academics in particular subjects areas. Nursing programmes that take this specialist approach to teaching are unusual in that most nursing programmes are taught by nurse academics, who draw on a considerable amount of clinical experience to inform their teaching. Early nursing programmes tended towards subject areas being seen as insular and isolated from the general nursing content. Students were often left to integrate subject specific content into the nursing content with the consequence that limited views of nursing developed. A move away from the subject specialist approach enabled nursing content to integrate and open up the different supporting areas so that they could be applied to a whole view of nursing and a whole view of the patient/client (Greaves, 1987). More recently, in recognition of the equal relationship of theory to practice, lecturer/practitioner's are used as part of the teaching team to ensure the currency of nurse education, especially in relation to the clinical component.

The interdisciplinary approach

Here, cultural components are introduced in conjunction with classes offered by departments of anthropology or social science. This interdisciplinary that approach fits well with nursing programmes which incorporate elements of interprofessional education into the curriculum. The need for closer collaboration between health and social-care professions is growing exponentially with national and international policies calling for enhanced collaboration, reduced duplication of effort in programme delivery, better use of resources, and the need to more effectively equip nurses with the skills required to meet the needs of patients/clients in ever more complex situations (World Health Organization, 1988; Department of Health, 1998). Interprofessional education (IPE) is seen as the vehicle for preparing practitioners to deliver improved collaboration. However, it is not without its problems for nurse educators. Limited literature around its use in pre-registration nursing programmes means that little is known of the impact this type of learning has on future professionals. Evaluation of such initiatives draws mostly on nursing programmes in the USA, and caution is needed if attempting to make generalisable conclusions from these studies to the UK (Reeves, 2000). In addition, limited methodological literature is available to nurse educators to inform IPE approaches within nursing programmes. Where IPE is a feature of programme delivery it is likely that departments outside nursing contribute to teaching as part of the strategy. The interdisciplinary approach to transcultural education, where cultural components are offered by departments such as social science, could facilitate IPE and enable nurse educators to study its effect on learning within UK nursing programmes.

The varieties of ways in which transcultural education can be included in the nursing curriculum indicate that no ideal approach exists. A 'one size fits all' approach is inappropriate as nurse education varies in much the same way as does transcultural education. When deciding what approach to take, consideration should be given to the practicalities of programme delivery, for example available programme time and whether the programme is pre- or post-registration (McGee, 1992). Another important consideration is the diversity of students on nursing programmes. In some localities the student population will be multicultural reflecting diversity within the local population. In other areas this will be less so. Teaching transcultural nursing requires recognition that differences exist within and between groups and not all students will react to transcultural nursing education in the same way. Educators may need to change the approach taken if it appears not to meet the needs of the students in developing cultural competence. Sensitivity to the reactions of others may require a flexible approach to teaching and learning about culture in the context of health-care practice.

Once a decision has been reached on how to incorporate transcultural education into the curriculum, be it integrated, unit-specific, or interdisciplinary, a decision is needed on the cultural content to be included in order for cultural competency to be achieved. Cultural competence is essential for nurses working in an ever-increasingly multicultural society. Campinha-Bacote (1994) writes that cultural competence is a process in which the health-care provider continuously strives to achieve the ability to work effectively within the cultural context of an individual or community from a diverse cultural or ethnic background. A number of models are available to guide curriculum content to ensure all relevant concepts and constructs are addressed. For the most part these focus on developing cultural competency.

Model for Developing Cultural Competence

Purnell's model

In order to assist nurses in the process of achieving cultural competency Purnell developed an organising framework for nurses to use as a cultural assessment tool, which has since developed into a model that can be used to promote cultural understanding about the human situation during times of illness, wellness, and health promotion (Purnell, 1998). His model is a conceptualisation from multiple theories, and a research base gained from organisational/administrative therapies, anthropology, sociology, anatomy and physiology, biology, psychology, religion, history, linguistics, nutrition, and the clinical practice settings in nursing and medicine. This model is complex. It is depicted as having an outer circle representing the global society, with an underlying second circle representing the community; a third inner circle represents the family, and an innermost circle represents the person. The inner section of the circle is divided into twelve interrelated cultural domains and their concepts. The centre of the circle remains empty to represent unknown aspects of the cultural group. The twelve cultural domains are heritage, communication, family roles, workforce issues, biocultural ecology, high-risk behaviours, nutrition, pregnancy and childbearing, death rituals, spirituality, health-care practices, and health-care practitioner concepts (for a detailed description read Purnell, 2000). The model has been used in practice, administration and research. However, our interest here is its use as an educational tool. Purnell describes the model as being acceptable for staff development and for use in academic settings by nurses, nutritionists, physicians, physical therapists, anthropologists, and social workers. Students in introductory lessons can use the model in its simplest form with no requirement for an in-depth understanding of conceptual models and theories to incorporate the model into practice. The model has also been used in an integrated nursing curriculum by including an overview of culture in an introductory module, followed by specific units that focus on selected domains. The Purnell model, originally developed in 1995, is subject to ongoing development. It has been translated into Spanish and French and used by nurses to guide the acquisition and practice of cultural competency in a variety of care delivery settings, in a number of countries. Although complex, the model does provide a detailed account of the kinds of issues and questions of relevance for nurses working in a multicultural society. Nurses need to be mindful of the cultural factors that impact on an individual's experience of health and illness. Purnell's model draws attention to culture and provides a framework to allow nurses to organise their practice to take account of cultural factors impacting on health and well-being. It facilitates inclusion of transcultural nursing into the curriculum in a meaningful way.

Campinha-Bacote's model

Campinha-Bacote (1999) created a model entitled The Process of Cultural Competence in the Delivery of Healthcare Services: A Culturally Competent Model of Care, with the aim to understand how to gain cultural competence. The model has been used in psychiatric nursing, rehabilitation nursing, and critical care nursing, but here we are interested in its use in nurse education. The model visually represents the components required for cultural competence, which are considered by Campinha-Bacote to be cultural awareness, cultural knowledge, cultural encounters, and cultural desire. Nurse educators can use these components to structure cultural content within the nursing curriculum. The model provides concrete explanations of the concept and process of cultural competence to guide nursing actions (Campinha-Bacote, 1999).

The first step for students towards achieving cultural competence is cultural awareness, which Campinha-Bacote describes as the process of becoming sensitive to interactions with other cultural or ethnic groups (Campinha-Bacote, 1995). By using the model as a framework, nurse educators can be guided to choose opportunities to increase students' cultural awareness in a variety of ways ranging from giving students a cultural values questionnaire, using cultural scenarios and role playing, or providing students with a cultural exchange experience. Whatever the method for increasing cultural awareness, students must be given the opportunity to discuss the activity and be supported in their efforts to use and express cultural attributes in the classroom without feeling uncomfortable or negatively different (Campinha-Bacote, 1998).

Cultural knowledge is the second step to achieving cultural competence. It involves acquiring a knowledge base of how others view the world. Within the nursing curriculum cultural content should aim to increase the students' knowledge base of specific issues such as stereotyping, discrimination, and racism as well as more general cultural content such as recognising difference within and between ethnic groups. Methods for delivering cultural knowledge may include classroom discussion, reading relevant literature including research, and using other sources such as film, music and art to increase cultural knowledge.

The third step to achieving cultural competence in Campinha-Bacote's model is cultural skill, which sees nurse educators encouraging students' to assess each patient/client individually in order to eradicate cultural assumptions made strictly on the basis of observation. The aim here is to move the student away from the notion that if someone looks the same as someone else then they are of the same cultural heritage and therefore have the same cultural beliefs. Cultural assessment tools can assist the process of guiding students towards achieving cultural skills. Whichever tool is used nurses should ensure that the nursing assessment is underpinned by knowledge of the patient/client's disease or disorder and knowledge of their cultural heritage. In so doing the patient/client's experience of ill health can be placed within the context of cultural background. Examples of cultural assessments applicable to different client groups can be found in Chapters *Three, Four, Five*, and *Six* of this book.

Cultural encounters make up the fourth stage of Campinha-Bacote's model. Here the student is involved in a direct interaction and is enabled to put the theory of transcultural nursing into practice. The role of the nurse educator is to provide appropriate opportunities for cultural encounters to take place. This may be relatively easy within some nursing programmes due to the diversity of local health service users. In other locations cultural encounters may be more difficult to experience. Alternatives to direct encounters may be facilitated by cultural exchange, which may involve working in partnership with other higher education institutions (HEIs) to provide opportunities for students to experience health-care practice in another locality, or even in another country if this is deemed appropriate. One such cultural exchange opportunity is Scholes and Moore's (2000) clinical exchange model for achieving culturally sensitive care, which incorporated a clinical exchange into a pre-registration European nursing degree. The degree programme, run by three collaborating institutions in England, the Netherlands, and Spain included common and shared learning, facilitated through two summer schools and the development of a second language. This was followed by a three-month clinical placement in one of the other 'base' institutions clinical environments. The exchange programme is underpinned by the belief that, in addition to learning about other cultures by exposure to ethnic groups within our own society, the process can be enhanced by total emersion into another culture for a period of no less than three months. It is argued that total emersion allows the student time to come to terms with that culture, by providing opportunities to work with staff as well as patients/clients from alternative cultural backgrounds (Williamson, 1994). Williamson (1994) argues that two important connections are triggered by immersing students into a different culture. First, students share a common profession, and second, students are thrust into an alternative culture where they themselves become the minority and thus experience disadvantage (struggling with another language, and working in a relatively strange environment). This is a powerful argument for exchange experience, in that in multicultural Great Britain it is likely to be the case that the nursing student belongs to the majority ethnic group and will struggle to experience the types of disadvantage being in the minority affords.

Scholes and Moore report the model as problematic in ways that are not surprising. Running a programme across the continent of Europe is complex due to the diverse mix of countries, languages, and dialects. Each country has its own framework for registration and education provision. While the European Communities Council has attempted to identify common theoretical outcomes to ensure parity of initial preparation, thereby increasing nurse mobility, the individual countries interpretation of these rules still leaves greater differences than commonalities (Scholes and Moore, 2000). In spite of the acknowledged difficulties, the authors report great pride in the programme, which ultimately seeks to promote a 'European dimension' to nursing through common and shared learning components. Furthermore, they envisage continuation of the model as a way of developing the nursing students' cultural awareness.

These findings from recent research by Cinnirella and Hamilton (2007) are worth considering for curriculum planners considering cultural exchange modules within nursing programmes. The researchers explored feelings of European identity, and attitudes towards Europe manifested in two groups within the British population. The indigenous white British population and the South Asian ethnic minority were surveyed using scales to evaluate British, European and ethnic identities and attitudes towards Europe. The indigenous white British respondents, who displayed a strong sense of national identity, negatively correlated with European identity. In contrast, the South Asian respondents displayed positive feelings of identification on all three levels, and a British identity that correlated positively with European identity. The research highlights the importance of avoiding making assumptions that students will react positively to cultural exchange, as attitudes towards ethnic identity are diverse and often deeply rooted in cultural history. If a model of cultural exchange is considered attention should be paid to where in the programme it should be located, how students are prepared for the experience, how the experience is evaluated, and the kinds of support students are given during and after the cultural exchange. It is also worth considering whether cultural exchange should be offered as a core or optional experience. Optional experiences, while giving the student the opportunity to 'opt out' if they do not wish to study in another county, for any reason (be it financial, personal or culturally determined) may lead to inconsistency of experience across the nursing programme as a whole. Inconsistency in experience has implications for the validity of programme evaluation.

Returning to the final stage for achieving cultural competence Campinha-Bacote's model discusses cultural desire, which involves having a true aspiration to work in diverse cultural settings. Cultural desire should include a willingness to include the patient/client's cultural rituals within the plan of care, as long as these are not harmful to the individual. In *Introduction* to this book we considered the comment made by Irena Papadopoulos who, when working in deprived multicultural area of London, learnt to respect the views and wishes of patients/clients who often used traditional, but unscientific ways to treat illnesses. Cultural desire requires that nurses respect the need for people from multiethnic backgrounds to be consulted about their care and to have their wishes incorporated into the care plan. When this is not possible, for example in emergency situations where decisions have to be made immediately, steps should be taken to ensure patients/clients and their carers fully understand the reasons for deviations from agreed care plans. Interpreters may be required to ensure that misunderstandings are avoided and to maintain the integrity of the relationship between patient/client and the professional. Nurse educators play an important role in fostering cultural desire by ensuring the quality of transcultural education within the nursing curriculum. Thought should be given to the most appropriate approach, choice of content, and choice of learning and teaching methods. Account should also be taken of the type of nursing programme and the diversity of students on the programme.

Conclusions

We have considered ways in which nurse educators can incorporate transcultural nursing into the curriculum. These include approaches such as an integrative approach, a unit-construction approach, a course approach, and an interdisciplinary approach. Whichever approach is taken, thought should be given to how the transcultural education fits with the nursing programme as a whole. To avoid a mismatch, the assumptions and philosophies underpinning the curriculum need to be consistent with those underpinning the approach to learning and teaching transcultural nursing. A number of models are available to guide curriculum planners in choosing content and learning/teaching methods. The choice of model should take into account the practicalities of delivering the content within the confines of the existing programme. Purnell's and Campinha-Bacote's models are useful tools for guiding nurse educators to the kinds of cultural content that should be included in the nursing curriculum.

With respect to the aims described earlier in this book, students and practitioners have been provided with a foundation to the theory and practice of transcultural nursing. A comprehensive guide to different cultures has not been provided, so for this, the reader is guided towards Leininger and McFarland's comprehensive text *Transcultural Nursing: Concepts, Theories, Research & Practice* (Leininger and McFarland, 2002). While this book addresses specific cultural issues as they relate to adults, children, and people with mental health issues or learning disabilities, in relation to how a culturally appropriate assessment might be undertaken; it has not attempted to provide a definitive guide to cultural issues within those client groups. To this end you might want to read Andrews and Boyle's book on *Transcultural Concepts in Nursing Care* (2003). We have touched upon some of the ways in which cultural competency can be achieved and considered models for doing so, a more detailed account of how practitioners can be enabled to become culturally competent is available in *Transcultural Health and Social Care: Development of Culturally Competent Practitioners* (Papadopoulos, 2006).

APPENDIX: UK CENSUS 2001

Categories of Ethnic Origins

Which of the following categories best describes your ethnic origin?

A. White

- English, Scottish, or Welsh ☐
- Irish ☐
- Any other White background .... ☐

B. Mixed

- White/Caribbean ☐
- White/African ☐
- White/Asian ☐
- Any other Mixed background .... ☐

C. Asian or Asian British

- Indian ☐
- Pakistani ☐
- Bangladeshi ☐
- Any other Asian background .... ☐

D. Black or Black British

- Caribbean ☐
- African ☐
- Any other Black background .... ☐

E. Chinese and other

- Chinese ☐
- Any other background .... ☐
- Ethnicity information refused ☐

References

Ahmad W (1993) *Race and Health in Contemporary Great Britain*. Open University Press: Buckingham (Chapter 2 pp.21–22).

Ahmad W (1994) Reflections on consanguinity and the birth outcome debate. *Journal of Public Health Medicine* **16**(4):423–438.

Ahmad W (1996) The trouble with culture. In: Kelleher D, Hillier S (eds) *Researching Cultural Differences in Health*. Routledge: London, pp. 190–219.

Ahmad W (2000) *Ethnicity, Disability and Chronic Illness*. Open University Press: Buckingham.

Ahmad W, Atkin K (1996) *'Race' and Community Care*. Open University Press: Buckingham.

Andrews MM, Boyle JS (2003) *Transcultural Concepts in Nursing Care*. Lippincott Williams & Wilkins: Philadelphia, PA.

Anionwu E, Atkin K (2001) *The Politics of Sickle cell and Thalassaemia*. Open University Press: Buckingham.

Atkin K (1996) An opportunity for change: voluntary sector provision in a mixed economy of care. In: Ahmad WIU, Atkin K (eds) *'Race and Community Care*. Open University Press: Buckingham, pp. 144–60.

Atkin K, Rollings J (1996) Looking after their own? Family care-giving among Asian and Afro–Caribbean communities. In: Ahmad WIU, Atkin K (eds) *'Race and Community Care*. Open University Press: Buckingham, pp. 73–86.

Baron-Cohen *et al.*, 1992[details needed].

Baron-Cohen S, Bolton P (1993) *Autism: The Facts*. Oxford University Press: Oxford, pp. 14–19

Barrot (1996) cited by Nazroo J (1999) The racialisation of ethnic inequalities in health. In: Dorling D, Simpson S (1999) *Statistics in Society*. Arnold: London, pp. 215–22.

Bayley J (1998) *Iris: A Memoir of Iris Murdock*. Gerald Duckworth: London.

Bennett MJ (1986) A developmental approach to training for intercultural sensitivity. *International Journal of Intercultural Relations* **10**(2):179–95.

Berlin EA, Fowkes WC (1983) A teaching framework for cross-cultural health care. *The Western Journal of Medicine* **139**(9):934–39.

Bieri D, Reeve RA, Champion GD, Addicoat L, Ziegler JB (1990) Cited by Henley A, Schott J (1999) *Culture, Religion and Patient Care in a Multi-Ethnic Society*. Age Concern England: London, p. 145.

Bowler I (1993) 'They're not the same as us': midwives' stereotypes of South Asian descent maternity patients. *Sociology of Health and Illness* **15**(2):157–178.

Bradby H (1995) Ethnicity and health: not a Black and White issue. *Sociology of Health and Illness* **17**(3):405–417.

Bradby H (2001) Communication, interpretation and translation. In: Culley L, Dyson SM (eds) *Ethnicity and Nursing Practice*. Palgrave: Basingstoke, pp. 129–48.

Bruner J.S. (1960) *The Process of Education*. Vintage Books, Random House: New York, NY.

Byerly E (1977) Teaching transcultural care: A guide for teachers of nursing and health care. In: McGee P (1992) *Testing the Water: Multicultural Education Today*. Chapman and Hall: London, pp. 15–16.

Campinha-Bacote J (1994) Cultural competence in psychiatric mental health nursing. A conceptual model. *Nursing Clinics of North America* **29**(1):108.

Campinha-Bacote J (1995) The quest for cultural competence in nursing care. *Nursing Forum* **30**(4):19–25.

Campinha-Bacote J (1998) Cultural diversity in nursing education: Issues and concerns. *Journal of Nursing Education* **37**(1):3–4.

Campinha-Bacote J (1999) A model and instrument for addressing cultural competence in health care. *Journal of Nursing Education* **38**(5):203–7.

Cavilli-Sforza LL, Menozzi P, Piazza A (1996) *The History and Geography of Human Genes* (abridged edition). Princeton University Press: Princeton, NJ.

Cinnirella M, Hamilton S (2007) Are all Britons reluctant Europeans? Exploring European identity and attitudes to Europe among citizens of South Asian ethnicity. *Ethnic and Racial Studies* **30**(3):481–501.

Cohen D, Eisdorfer C (2001) *The Loss of Self: A Family Resource for the Care of Alzheimer's Disease and Related Diseases*. WW Norton & Amp: New York, NY.

Culley L (2001) Nursing, culture and competence. In: Culley L, Dyson SM (eds) *Ethnicity and Nursing Practice*. Palgrave: Basingstoke, pp. 109–127.

Culley L, Dyson SM (2001) *Ethnicity and Nursing Practice*. Palgrave: Basingstoke.

Culley L, Dyson SM, Ham-Ying S, Young W (2001) Caribbean nurses and racism in the NHS in Culley L, Dyson SM (eds) *Ethnicity and Nursing Practice*.Palgrave: Basingstoke, pp. 231–49.

Department for Education and Skills (2004) *Every Child Matters: Change for Children*. DES: London.

Department of Health (1998) *A First Class Service: Quality in the NHS*. HMSO: London.

Department of Health (2001) *Valuing People: A New Strategy for Learning Disability for the 21st Century*. Cm 5086. DH: London.

Dick M (2007) UK Forum on Haemoglobin Disorders. NHS Sickle Cell and Thalassaemia Screening Programme in Partnership with the Sickle Cell Society: London.

Dyer R (1997) *White*. Routledge: London.

Dyson SE (2005a) Global boarders: Leaving Zimbabwe – factors influencing undergraduate students' decision to study nursing in the UK. In: Yfantopoulos J, Papanikos G (eds) (2005) *Health Economics Management and Policy.* Atiner: Athens, pp. 135–72.

Dyson SM (2005b) *Ethnicity and Screening for Sickle Cell/Thalassaemia: Lessons for Practice from the Voices of Experience.* Elsevier: London.

Dyson SM, Smaje C (2001) The health status of minority ethnic groups. In: Culley L, Dyson SM (eds) *Ethnicity and Nursing Practice.* Palgrave: Basingstoke, pp. 39–65.

Fadiman A (1997) *The Sprit Catches You and You Fall Down.* Farrar, Straus and Giroux: New York, NY.

Fernando S (1995) *Mental Health in a Multi-Ethnic Society.* Routledge: London.

France-Dawson M (1990) Sickle cell conditions and health knowledge. *Nursing Standard* **4**(5):30–34.

Frith U, Soares I (1993) Research into the earliest detectable signs of autism: what the parents say. *Communication* 1993; **27**(3):17–18.

Fryer P (1984) *Staying Power: The History of Black People in Great Britain.* Pluto Press: London.

Gaines AD (1992) *Ethno-Psychiatry: The Cultural Construction of Professional and Folk Psychiatries.* State University of New York Press: Albany, NY.

Geldmacher DS (2001) *Contemporary Diagnosis and Management of Alzheimer's Disease.* Associates in Medical Marketing: Newtown, PA.

Gerrish K (1997) Preparation of nurses to meet the needs of an ethnically diverse society: educational implications. *Nurse Education Today* **17**:359–65.

Gerrish K, Husband C, Mackenzie J (1996a) *Nursing for a Multi-Ethnic Society.* Open University Press: Buckingham.

Gerrish K, Husband C, Mackenzie J (1996b) Ethnicity, the minority ethnic community and health care delivery. In: Ahmad WIU, Husband C (eds) *Race, Health and Social Care.* Open University Press: Buckingham.

Gerrish K, Husband C, Mackenzie J (1997) Preparation of nurses to meet the needs of an ethnically diverse society: educational implications. *Nurse Education Today* **17**(5): 359–65.

Giger J, Davidhizar R (1998) Educating the culturally diverse healthcare student. *Nurse Educator* **23**(2):38–42.

Gillberg C (1990) Autism and pervasive development disorders. *Journal of Child Psychology and Psychiatry* **31**(1):99–119.

Glover I, Bellwood S (2004) *Southeast Asia: From Prehistory to History.* Routledge: London.

Greaves F (1987) *The Nursing Curriculum: Theory and Practice.* Croom Helm: London.

Grundy SM (1999) Primary Prevention of Coronary Heart Disease: Integrating Risk Assessment with Intervention. *Circulation* **100**:988–98.

Haddon M (2004) *The Curious Incident of the Dog in the Night Time* (adult edition). Red Fox, Random House: London.

Hage G (1998) *White Nation: Fantasies of White Supremacy in a Multicultural Society.* Pluto Press Australia: Annandale NSW.

Henley A (1982) *Caring for Muslims and their Families: Religious Aspects of Care.* National Extension College: Cambridge.

Henley A, Schott J (1999) *Culture, Religion and Patient Care in a Multi-Ethnic Society.* Age Concern England: London.

Hogston R (2002) Managing nursing care. In: Hogston R, Simpson P (eds) *Foundations of Nursing Practice: Making the Difference*. Palgrave Macmillan: London.

Holland K, Hog C (2001) *Cultural Awareness in Nursing and Health Care*. Arnold: London.

Home Office (2002a) *The Migrant Population in the UK: Fiscal Effects*. The Home Office: London.

Home Office (2002b) *Migrants in the UK: Their Characteristics and Labour Market Outcomes and Impacts*. The Home Office: London.

Humphries J (2007) *Autism: recognising the signs in young children*. National Autistic Society (Surrey Branch). http://www.mugsy.org/pmh.htm/.

Johnson MRD (2001) Ethnic monitoring and nursing. In: Culley L, Dyson SM (eds) *Ethnicity and Nursing Practice*. Palgrave: Basingstoke.

Kavanagh KH (2003) Transcultural perspectives in mental health nursing. In: Andrews MM, Boyle JS (2003) *Transcultural Concepts in Nursing Care*. Lippincott Williams & Wilkins: Philadelphia, pp. 272–314.

Kershen A (2005) *Strangers, Aliens, and Asians: Huguenots, Jews, and Bangladeshis in Spitalfields 1660–2000*. Routledge: London.

Kim YY (1992) Intercultural communication competence: a systems theoretic view. In: Gudykunst WB, Kimm YY (eds) *Readings on Communication with Strangers*. McGraw-Hill: New York, NY.

Kincheloe JL, Steinberg SR, Rodriguez NM, Chennault RE (1998) *White Reign: Deploying Whiteness in America*. St Martin's Griffin, New York, NY.

Kulwicki A (1996) Cited by Henley A, Schott J (1999) *Culture, Religion and Patient Care in a Multiethnic Society.* Age Concern England: London.

Leininger M (1995) *Transcultural Nursing. Concepts, Theories, Research and Practices* (2nd edn). John Wiley: New York, NY.

Leininger M, McFarland M (2002) *Transcultural Nursing: Concepts, Theories, Research and Practice* (3rd edn). McGraw Hill: New York, NY (p. 120).

Levy A (2004) *Small Island*. Headline: London.

Mace N, Rabbins P (2001) *The 36-Hour Day: A Family Guide for Caring with Persons with Alzheimer Disease, Reacted Dementing Illnesses, and Memory Loss in Later Life*. Warner Books: New York, NY.

MacPherson W (1999) *The Stephen Lawrence Inquiry: Report of an Inquiry by Sir William MacPherson*. Cm 4262-I. The Stationery Office: London.

Mason D (1995) *Race and Ethnicity in Modern Great Britain*. Oxford University Press: Oxford.

McEwan G, Kelsey J, Richardson J, Glasper A (2003) Insights into child and family health. In: Grandis S, Long G, Glasper A, Jackson P (eds) *Foundation Studies for Nursing. Using Enquiry-Based Learning*. Palgrave Macmillan: London.

McGee P (1992) *Teaching Transcultural Care; A Guide for Teachers of Nursing and Health Care*. Chapman and Hall: London.

McReady N (2003) Prompt intervention may slow Alzheimer's decline. *British Medical Journal* 7 June: 1232.

Melzack R (1975) The McGill pain questionnaire: major properties and scoring methods. *Pain*, **1**:277–99.

Meremikwu M (2006) Sickle cell disease. *Clinical Evidence* **15**:1–3.

Michalik U, Konopnicka M (2007) *Polish people apart: Eastern immigration: Why go West?* Rising East Online. http://ueldirect-b.uel.ac.uk/risingeast/currentissue/academic/urszula.htm.

Millennium Charter (2000) *Action for Sick Children*. http://www.actionforsickchildren.org/.

Mir G (2007) Transcultural health-care practice: Core practice module 4: Ethnicity and learning disabilities; Section 3: Planning better services. In: Husband C, Torri B (eds) *Transcultural Health Care Practice: An Educational Resource For Nurses And Health Care Practitioners*. http://www.rcn.org.uk/resources/transcultural/learningdisability/.

Modood T (1998) Anti-essentialism, multiculturalism and the 'recognition' of religious groups. *The Journal of Political Philosophy* **6**(4):378–99.

Narayanasamy A (2003) Transcultural nursing: how do nurses respond to cultural needs? *British Journal of Nursing* **12**(2): pp. 36–45.

National Autistic Society (1997) *Statistics Sheet. How Many People Have Autistic-Spectrum Disorder?* National Autistic Society: London.

Nazroo J (1997) T*he Health of Great Britain's Ethnic Minorities*. Policy Studies Institute: London.

Nazroo J (1999) The racialisation of ethnic inequalities in health. In: Dorling D, Simpson S (eds) *Statistics in Society*. Arnold: London, pp. 215–22.

Nursing and Midwifery Council (2002) *Code of Professional Conduct*. NMC: London.

Papadopoulos I (2002) Meeting health-care needs in culturally diverse societies. In: Daly J, *et al*. (eds) *Contexts of Nursing: An Introduction*. Blackwell Science: Oxford.

Papadopoulos I (ed) (2006) *Transcultural Health and Social Care: Development of Culturally Competent Practitioners*. Elsevier: Edinburgh.

Papadopoulos I, Lees S (2002) Developing culturally competent researchers. *Journal of Advanced Nursing* **37**(3):258–64.

Pearson A, Vaughan B, FitzGerald M (1996) *Nursing Models for Practice*. Butterworth Heinemann: London.

Petersen S, Peto V, Rayner M (2004) Coronary heart disease statistics. British Heart Foundation Health Promotion Research Group. Department of Public Health. University of Oxford: Oxford.

Policy Research on Ageing and Ethnicity (2005) cited by Sims JM (2007) *The Vietnamese Community in Great Britain – Thirty Years On*. The Runnymede Trust: London.

Purnell L (2000) A description of the Purnell model for cultural competence. *Journal of Transcultural Nursing* **11**(1):40–46.

Purnell L, Paulanka B J (1998) *Transcultural Health Care. A Culturally Competent Approach*. FA Davis: Philadelphia, PA.

Quality Assurance Agency (2001) Benchmark Statement Healthcare Programmes: Nursing. Quality Assurance Agency for Higher Education: London, pp. 6–17.

Race Relations Act (1976) (Statutory Duties) Order 2001. HMSO: London.

Race Relations Amendment Act (2000) HMSO: London.

Rajamanickam B (2007) Transcultural health-care practice: Core practice module 5: Mental health and minority ethnic groups. In: Husband C, Torri B (eds) *Transcultural Health Care Practice: An Educational Resource For Nurses And Health Care Practitioners*. http://www.rcn.org.uk/resources/transcultural/learningdisability/.

Reeves S (2000) Community-based inter-professional education for medical, nursing and dental students. *Health and Social Care in the Community* **8**(4):269–76.

Roper N, Logan W, Tierney A (1983) *Using a Model for Nursing*. Churchill Livingstone: Edinburgh.

Rose S, Lewontin R, Kamin L (1984) *Not In Our Genes: Biology, Ideology and Human Nature*. Penguin: Harmondsworth.

Runnymede Trust (2000) Reappraising the Corporate Face in Europe. No. 321. The Runnymede Bulletin March 2000, pp. 1–28.

Sarafino EP (1990) Health psychology. *Biopsychosocial Interactions*. John Wiley and Sons: New York, NY.

Sarjeant GR, Sarjeant BE (2001) *Sickle Cell Disease* (3rd edn). Oxford University Press: Oxford.

Scholes J, Moore D (2000) Clinical exchange: one model to achieve culturally sensitive care. *Nursing Inquiry* **7**:61–71.

Serrant-Green L (2001) Transcultural nursing education: a view from within. *Nurse Education Today* **21**: 670–78.

Sheldon T, Parker H (1992) Race and ethnicity in health research. *Journal of Public Health Medicine* **14**(2):104–10.

Sims JM (2007) *The Vietnamese Community in Great Britain – Thirty Years On*. The Runnymede Trust: London.

Smaje C (1996) Cited in Culley L, Dyson S (eds) (2001) *Ethnicity and Nursing Practice*. Palgrave: Buckingham, p. 110.

Smith GD, Chaturvedi N, Harding S, Nazroo J, Williams R (2000) Ethnic inequalities in health: a review of UK epidemiological evidence. *Critical Public Health* **10**(4), 375–408.

Taba H (1962) The concept of the curriculum. Cited in: Greaves F (1987) *The Nursing Curriculum: Theory and Practice*. Croom Helm: London.

Wheeler DK (1967) The concept of the curriculum. Cited in: Greaves F (1987) *The Nursing Curriculum: Theory and Practice*. Croom Helm: London, pp. 1–8.

Wild S, McKeigue P (1997) Cross-sectional analysis of mortality by country of birth in England and Wales. *British Medical Journal* **314**:705–10.

Williamson J (1994) cited by Scholes J, Moore D (2000) Clinical exchange: one model to achieve culturally sensitive care. *Nursing Inquiry* **7**:61–71.

Wing (1980) Childhood autism and social class: a question of selection? *British Journal of Psychiatry* **137**, 410–17.

World Health Organization (1988) *Learning Together to Work Together.* WHO: Geneva.

Useful web sites

1990 Trust
http://www.blink.org.uk/

Action for Sick Children
http://http://www.actionforsickchildren.org/

Afiya Trust
http://www.afiya-trust.org/

Black and Asian History map
http://www.channel4.com/history/microsites/B/blackhistorymap/

Commission for Racial Equality
http://www.cre.gov.uk/

Department for Education and Skills
http://www.everychildmatters.gov.uk/

Department of Health
http://www.doh.gov.uk/race_equality/

Diversiton: Respecting diversity in the workplace
http://www.diversiton.com/

EuroTalk Interactive
http://www.eurotalk.co.uk/

Human Rights Act 1998
http://www.dca.gov.uk/peoples-rights/human-rights/

Immigration, Work Visa and Work Permit Services
http://www.workpermit.com/

Institute for Race Relations
http://www.irr.org.uk/

Joint Council for the Welfare of Immigrants
http://www.jcwi.org.uk/

Kings Fund (London)
http://www.kingsfund.org.uk/eLibrary/assets/applets/Ethheorg.pdf/

Local Interfaith Guide
http://www.interfaith.org.uk/

National Autistic Society (Surrey Branch)
http://www.mugsy.org/pmh.htm/

Refugee Council
http://www.refugeecouncil.org.uk/

Religious Calendars
http://www.support4learning.org.uk/shap/index.htm/

Rising East Online
http://www.uel.ac.uk/risingeast/

Royal College of Nursing Transcultural Healthcare Practice
http://www.rcn.org.uk/resources/transcultural/

Runnymede Trust
http://www.runnymedetrust.org/

Sickle Cell Screening
http://www.screening.nhs.uk/sickleandthal/

Sickle Cell Society
http://www.sicklecellsociety.org/